ESSENTIAL OILS

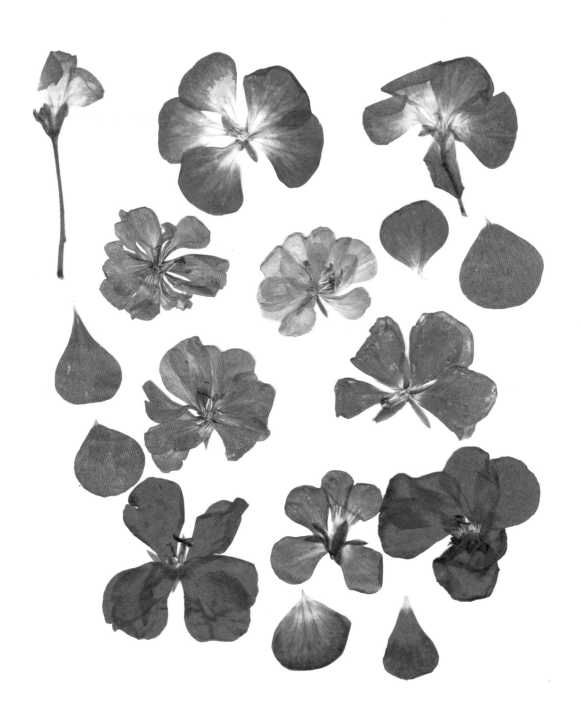

ESSENTIAL OILS

YOUR AROMATHERAPY GUIDE
TO AYURVEDIC HEALING

DR RAVI RATAN

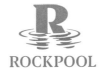

ROCKPOOL

A Rockpool book
PO Box 252
Summer Hill, NSW 2130
Australia
rockpoolpublishing.co
Follow us! **f** ⊙ rockpoolpublishing
Tag your images with #rockpoolpublishing

ISBN 978-1-925924-57-2

Cover by Tracy Loughlin, Rockpool Publishing
Typesetting by Jessica Le, Rockpool Publishing

Printed and bound in China
10 9 8 7 6 5 4 3 2 1

A catalogue record for this
book is available from the
National Library of Australia

Aromatherapy is a complementary therapy, without any side effects when used correctly. It is recommended to consult your doctor or therapist before using aromatherapy to replace or in conjunction with any ongoing medication. The author and publishers disclaim all responsibility for any adverse reaction caused by inappropriate use of or poor quality essential oils.

ABOUT THE AUTHOR

Dr Ravi Ratan is a leading aromatherapist based in India. He is descended from a long line of healers and teachers, who inspired him to become a healer, too. As well as holding two Masters degrees, Dr Ratan has a Doctorate of Science (Medicina Alternativa) from the Open International University of Alternative Medicine.

After working for more than thirty years in the perfume industry, Dr Ratan discovered the healing potential of natural essential oils. Aromatherapy became his passion, especially the healing and therapeutic potential of essential oils on a physical as well as psychological level. Motivated by his successful results in healing and healthcare, Dr Ratan has focused on complete body therapy.

Dr Ravi Ratan has undertaken extensive clinical research work on the use of essential oils for health and healing, and has created an aromatherapy workout regimen for the physical body focusing on problem areas and identifying causes and aromatherapy solutions. He now trains beauticians, alternative therapists and health club professionals in his methods.

In his aromatherapy practice, Dr Ratan combines ancient Ayurvedic wisdom with modern aromatherapy principles – Vedic Aromatherapy – and creates unique blends for health and healing. Prominent among these are his anointments for seven chakras (the body's energy centres), which have been found very effective in restoring the healthy balance of mind, body and spirit. They have been used effectively by Dr Ratan's wife, Minoo Ratan, a practising psycho-aromatherapist and healer, in the treatment of psychosomatic disorders and other chronic conditions. Thus, the fundamentals of five elements and three gunas (properties) have been used to select various essential oils for chakra healing and balancing.

Both Ravi and Minoo Ratan have done extensive healing work in Vedic aromatherapy, using essential oils for chakra energising and harmonising, and together they wrote *Journey Through the Chakras*. They have received extensive media coverage.

As well as therapies and healing including emotional release work, Dr Ratan conducts regular training programs and workshops in Aromatherapy (Basic and Advanced), Chakras and Crystals Healing, and Aroma Massages with Manual Lymphatic Drainage (MLD) in the USA, UK, Australia, India, Canada and Dubai.

Dr Ratan can be found at www.aromatantra.com

This book is dedicated to my father, the late Dr Sushil Kumar Sharma,
renowned physician and surgeon from Muzaffarnagar, UP, India.
I always admired his healing touch and dedication to his profession.
While assisting him at his clinic during vacations, I saw him working on
non-healing ulcers, bedsores and gangrenous wounds. I wish he would
have looked at the healing powers of essential oils. It is his blessing
that I can now use essential oils in healing all these conditions.
He has always been a source of inspiration.

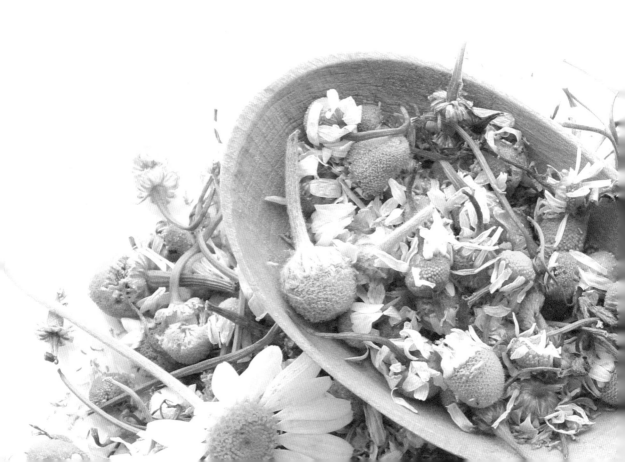

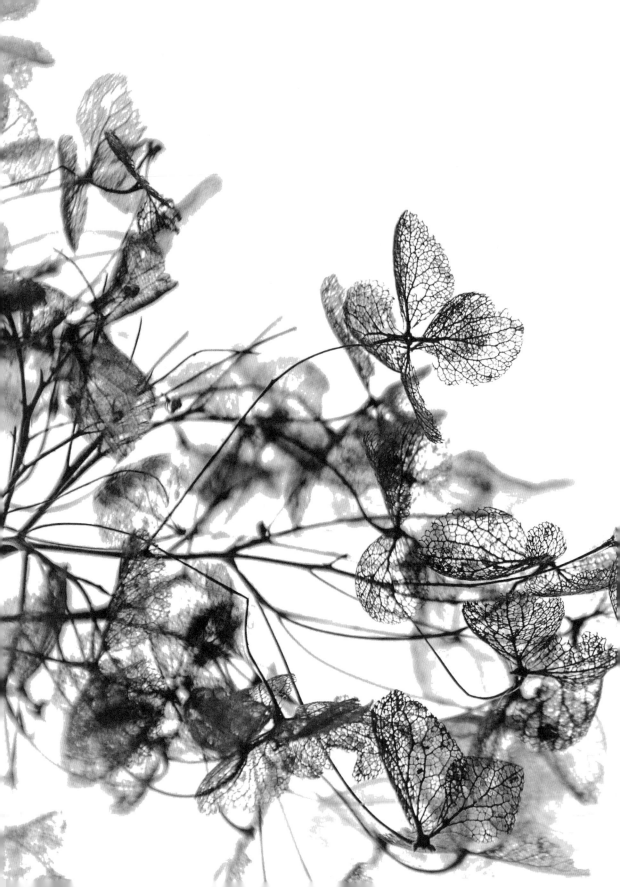

CONTENTS

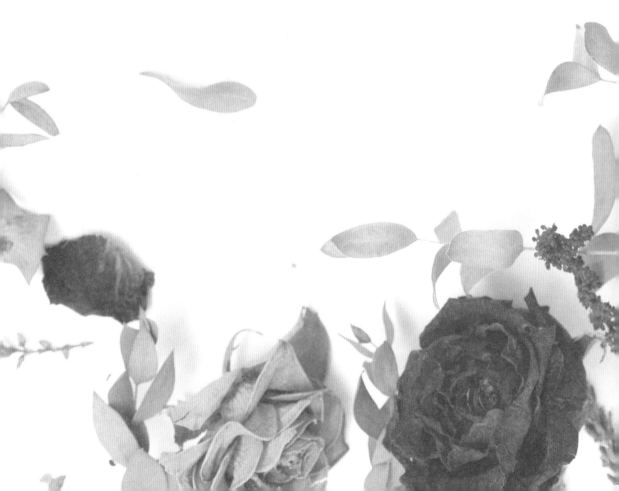

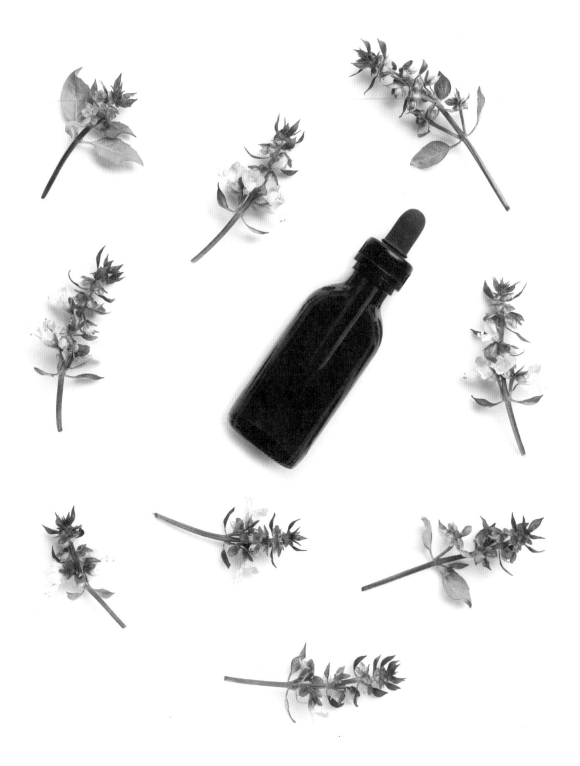

FOREWORD

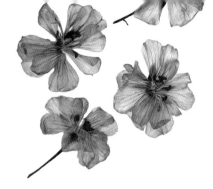

'That which cures is medicine;
that which heals is therapy.'
– Dr Minoo Ratan

Today, the world over, alternative and complementary therapies are being re-invoked and re-established to enable humankind to regain lost healthfulness. Aromatherapy is one of the safest and most effective complementary therapies, which can be used in conjunction with almost all other therapies and systems of healing. It works on us at physical, physiological and psychological levels.

Most human ailments begin in the mind. Psychosomatic disorders (PSD) are responsible for a great share of sales of over-the-counter medications, mainly for stress, anxiety and depression. Psychotherapy harmonises the agonised mind while aromatherapy acts as a support system for the mind as well as the diseased physical body and physiology. Empirical studies with aromatherapy have shown that it is most effective in increasing the body's immune system, ensuring that patients regain the confidence to fight back. The essential oils used in aromatherapy provide the necessary support to the immune system, since all essential oils are therapeutic in nature. Most are antiseptic, antibacterial and antiviral, while some are anti-fungal, rejuvenating, hormone-balancing, diuretic or have other specialised properties.

Coming from a family of medical practitioners, I have always been interested in healing and my interest in the mystical world of essential oils has grown each time they have given a result better than expected. Some of my clients have called these results 'miraculous', especially for the treatment of chronic conditions like bedsores, non-healing ulcers, and in postoperative recovery. Meanwhile my wife, Dr Minoo, a practising psycho-aromatherapist, has given me feedback on various formulations I've prepared for her patients, mainly for the treatment of psychosomatic disorders. *Essential Oils* contains not only our experience in the treatment of disorders, but also a sprinkle from a range of students in the field of health and healing.

Another dimension of essential oils I have explored is their use with Ayurvedic principles for healing and balancing the chakras. The chakra anointments I have created using the elements and gunas (properties) of the plants can also be used for treating physical, physiological and psychosomatic disorders.

This book provides comprehensive knowledge to enhance the understanding of beginners as well as professionals. It has been divided into four main parts. Part I covers the materia medica (the essential and carrier oils) in detail, followed by Part II on aromatherapy applications and methods of use. Part III is devoted to aromatic body and beauty therapy including how to take a case history and how to analyse the conditions to be focused on. For convenience and understanding, this section covers each part of the body (head to toe) separately, covering the problems, causes and aromatherapy solutions for each. Part IV covers the treatment of common ailments. Finally, the appendixes include detailed information on evening primrose oil, a ready reference guide to the therapeutic uses of essential oils and a handy glossary of terms.

I am delighted to share my knowledge and experience with my readers with this new edition.

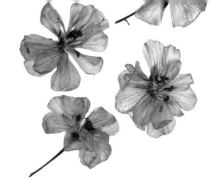

PART I

WHAT
IS
AROMATHERAPY?

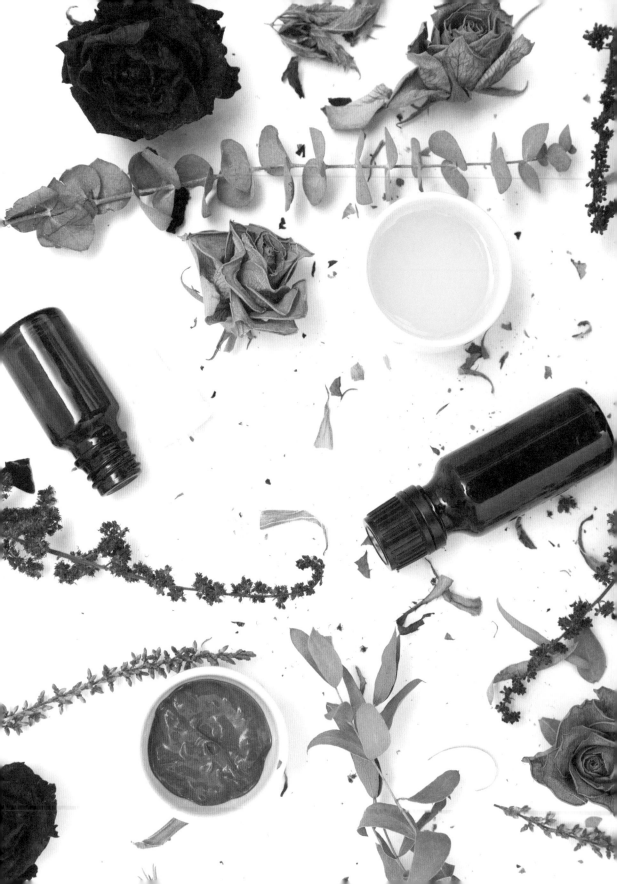

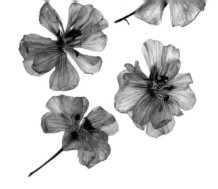

UNDERSTANDING AROMATHERAPY

Aromatherapy is the use of aromatic essences or oils extracted from plants for therapeutic purposes. Derived from the Greek word meaning 'spice', today the word 'aroma' is used more broadly to mean 'fragrance'. 'Therapy' means curative treatment. However 'aromatherapy' is a misnomer, giving the impression that the therapy works only by the sense of smell, whereas it also works by skin absorption, for example, when an essential oil is added to a carrier (such as a cream or lotion) for topical application.

Aromatherapy is a form of complementary medicine, like herbalism or Ayurveda, which draws on the healing powers of the plant world. However, instead of using the whole or a specific part of the plant, it employs only its essential oils. In Indian mythology, Lord Vishnu is the sustainer of the universe. One of his forms is Dhanwantri, the supreme Vaidya (physician). He propagated three forms of medicine: *churan* (medicine in solid form, such as a powder mix or *vatis*/tablets), medicine in liquid form (herbal extracts, tisanes, etc.) and medicine in gaseous form (plant essential oils, which are highly volatile and start evaporating when exposed to air). It is the medicine in gaseous form that forms the basis of modern aromatherapy. In Ayurvedic practice, the essential oils are the most potent of the three medications and usually administered to treat severe and chronic conditions.

Plant essential oils are a complex synergistic mix of organic chemicals with varied therapeutic effects. This makes an essential oil or a combination of essential oils versatile in their therapeutic effect, working at a physical, physiological and psychological level.

Aromatherapy can be used on two levels: aesthetic and medical. Aesthetically it can be used for skin, hair and beauty care as well as massage, daily wellbeing, natural fragrance and environmental cleansing and disinfecting. Medically it can be used to relieve physical, physiological and psychological imbalances. The advantage is that it can be used in conjunction with traditional medicine and all other therapeutic practices or healing work.

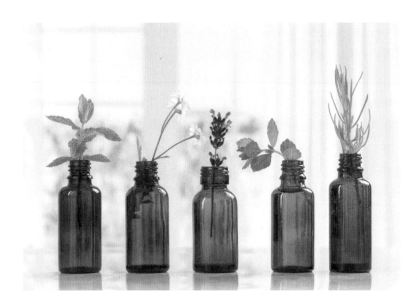

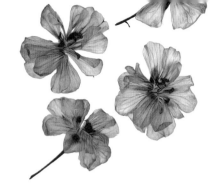

HISTORY AND ORIGIN OF AROMATHERAPY

Humans have always been dependent on the nutritional and therapeutic value of the plant world and the use of plants to cure diseases is as old as the human race itself. Animals, too, seek out particular herbs or grasses when they are unwell. Aromatic substances also played important roles in the medicinal practices of the Hebrew, Arabic and Indian civilisations. In the Indian epic *Ramayana,* a herb called Sanjeevani booti was administered to Laxman, the younger brother of Lord Ram, by crushing the leaves. When he inhaled the released aroma, Laxman revived after falling unconscious during the great battle with Ravana.

As mentioned earlier, the ancient Indian healing science of Ayurveda also uses plant essential oils; the difference is that aromatherapy uses the essential oils only while in Ayurveda the whole or part of the plant are also used.

The ancient Egyptians used aromatherapy as a way of life. At about the time the Chinese were developing acupuncture, the Egyptians were using aromatic oils and balsamic substances in both religious rituals and medicine. Records dating back to 4500 BC tell of perfumed oils, scented barks and resins, spices, aromatic vinegars, wines and beers used in medicine, ritual, astrology and embalming. The famous Egyptian art of embalming has echoes of today's aromatherapy principles. The embalmers knew of the natural antiseptic and antibiotic properties of plants and how these could be utilised in the process of preserving human bodies. Traces of resins like galbanum, frankincense and myrrh along with spices like clove, cinnamon and nutmeg have been isolated from the bandages of mummies. When Tutankhamen's tomb was opened in 1922, many pots were found containing substances such as myrrh and frankincense (both derived from tree resins). These were used medicinally as well as for making perfume, the two being interchangeable at that time.

Translations of hieroglyphics inscribed on papyri and stelae found in the Temple of Edfu (built between 237–57 BC) indicate that aromatic substances were blended to specific formulations by high priests and alchemists to make perfumes and medicinal potions. The priests knew of the power of certain odours to raise the spirits or promote tranquillity. A favourite perfume of the time was *kyphi*, a mixture of sixteen different essences – including myrrh and juniper – which was inhaled to heighten the senses and spiritual awareness of the priests. The incenses used in contemporary religious rituals serve much the same purpose.

While the Egyptians perfected the art of using the essences of plants to control emotion, putrefaction and disease, new discoveries about the medicinal power of plants were being made elsewhere. The Greeks developed medicine from part-superstition to science. Hippocrates (470–360 BC), popularly known as the father of modern medicine, was the first physician to base medical knowledge and treatment on accurate observation. One of his beliefs, that a daily aromatic bath and scented massage were a way to health, is the central principle of today's aromatherapy. Hippocrates was aware of the antibacterial properties of certain plants and when an epidemic of plague broke out in Athens he urged the people to burn aromatic plants at the corners of the street to protect themselves and prevent the plague from spreading.

This was a time when botanical knowledge was expanding, reaching its peak in the *Historia plantarum* (*Enquiry into Plants*) of Theophrastus (c. 371–287 BC), the so-called Father of Botany. At this time, there were 'immigrant' Greek physicians and seekers of knowledge who dominated the medical world. One of these was Dioscorides, a Greek surgeon in Nero's army, who between 70 and 50 BC wrote *De Materia Medica* (*On Medical Material*), one of the most comprehensive textbooks on the properties and uses of medicinal plants. He recorded details such as when a plant and its active principles might be at its most powerful. This indisputable fact of plant life, depending on time of day, time of the year and state of development, is utilised by the essential oil industry today. For instance, the poppy's yield in the morning is four times greater than in the evening. Jasmine's perfume and therefore the powers of its oil are strongest in the evening; this is why jasmine flowers are still picked at night in India for their aromatic properties.

The Romans, who were more interested in the culinary properties of plants than the medical, had enormous influence in the field of botany. Many herbal plants including parsley, fennel and lovage were introduced to Britain by the Romans. The middle ages in Europe (from approximately the sixth century to the Renaissance in the fourteenth century) was not an inspired period in terms of medical advancements. The sixteenth and seventeenth centuries were the times of the great herbals in Europe, when knowledge grew in leaps and bounds, with the founding of the Royal Society in Britain in 1663. Alongside this was the growth of a scientific approach to medicine, although belief in the therapeutic principles of essential oils co-existed. By the end of the eighteenth century, essential oils were widely used in medicine. Once chemistry began to flourish as a discipline and plant cures could be synthesised in the laboratory – cures that were stronger and faster in action – aromatherapy and its oils began to lose their place in pharmacopeia.

AROMATHERAPY IN THE TWENTIETH CENTURY

Dr Rene Maurice Gattefosse, a French perfumery scientist, is credited with the reincarnation of aromatherapy as a form of medicine, coining the term *Aromatherapie*, when he published a book by the same name in 1937 to describe the therapeutic action of aromatic plant essences. He explained at length the properties of essential oils and their methods of application, with examples of their antiseptic, bactericidal, antiviral and anti-inflammatory properties. He described how in 1910, after burning his hand in the laboratory, he plunged the hand into the nearest container, which happened to contain essential oil of lavender. He was astonished to find how quickly the pain ceased and the skin healed.

In association with a medical practitioner, Dr Jean Valnet, Dr Gattefosse continued to experiment with essential oils such as thyme, clove, chamomile and lemon, using men in the military hospital as his subjects during the First World War, with astounding results. Later the work was continued by Dr Valnet, who had to resort to the use of essential oils due to a shortage of antibiotics during the Second World War. Dr Valnet was a holder of the Légion d'honneur and founded the Société française de phytothérapie et d'aromathérapie, of which he was also the president. He published *The Practice of Aromatherapy* in 1980.

Until the Second World War, essential oils of cinnamon, clove, lemon, thyme and chamomile were used as natural disinfectants and antiseptics to fumigate hospital wards and sterilise instruments used in surgery and dentistry. The contemporary use of mainly cold-pressed vegetable oils as carriers for essential oils was introduced by French biochemist Marguerite Maurey, who was married to an Austrian homeopath. After extensive study of the absorption of essential oils through the skin, she recommended the use of vegetable oils as the carriers in aromatherapy. She extended the scope of her work, bringing aromatherapy into the world of aesthetics and cosmetology, allying medicine, health and beauty.

AROMATHERAPY TODAY

Aromatherapy is now widely practised and accepted in America, Europe, Britain and all developed countries, along with other forms of alternative medicine, collectively known as complementary systems of healing. Due to the side effects of synthetic drugs, the medicinal world is turning once again to natural remedies and healing practices. Using a synthetic drug to kill harmful bacteria is like cracking a nut with a sledgehammer: not only do they kill the harmful bacteria, they also destroy beneficial bacteria present in the body. Natural remedies such as essential oils, on the other hand, may act slowly in an antibiotic sense but while killing off the bacteria they also raise the body's immune system to strengthen its resistance to further attack. At the same time, they help the system rejuvenate itself, which is one of the most positive long-term effects of essential oils. The beneficial effect essential oils can have on the mind gives an added dimension to their use in healing.

All essential oils help to balance emotions to some degree and individually they may be noted for their stimulating, uplifting, relaxing or euphoric properties. At a psychological level, they can revive a tired mind and stimulate the memory. Interestingly, the area of the brain associated with smell is also that in which the memory is stored and aromas have been effectively used to stimulate the minds of those suffering from amnesia. Essential oils also increase our finest vibrations and assist the subtle body. They can stimulate and assist in the process of awakening, healing and opening the chakras, and strengthening the aura. To understand that aspect of essential oils we have to incorporate the Ayurvedic and tantric dimensions.

Observations of the effectiveness of essential oils are gradually being backed by studies taking place in parts of Central Europe, the USA, Australia and the UK. All essential oils appear to be antiseptic and bactericidal to some degree and some may also be helpful in the treatment of viral infections that are resistant to all known orthodox medicines. Many essential oils have the potential to stimulate healthy cell renewal and growth, and to regulate and restore the balance of the mind and body systems. Essential oils are noted, too, for their ability to reduce stress and stimulate sluggish circulation. These qualities, combined with their regenerative powers, give strength to claims that they boost the immune system.

With the renewed interest in natural and complementary therapies, essential oils offer a new approach to holistic health and healing beyond beauty and spa treatments, in particular as a way to good health or rehabilitation therapy.

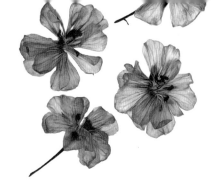

NATURE OF ESSENTIAL OILS

Essential oils are the odoriferous liquid components of plants. They influence growth and reproduction, attract pollinating insects, repel predators and protect the plant from disease. Unlike 'fixed' or fatty oils, they are highly volatile, which means they evaporate if exposed to the air. Many essences have the consistency of water or alcohol, including lavender, chamomile and rosemary. Others, such as myrrh and vetiver, are viscous, or thick and sticky, and still others, such as the exquisite rose otto, are semi-solid at room temperature but become liquid with the slightest warmth.

Essential oils are stored in tiny oil glands or sacs which are concentrated in different parts of the plant. They may be found in the petals (rose), leaves (eucalyptus), roots of grass (vetiver), heartwood (sandalwood), rind of the fruit (lemon), seeds (caraway), rhizomes (ginger) and sometimes in more than one part of the plant. Lavender, for instance, yields oil from both the flowers and the leaves, while the orange tree produces three differently scented essences with varying therapeutic properties: the heady bittersweet neroli (flower blossom) and a similar though less refined essence of petitgrain (leaves) and the cheery orange (rind/skin of the fruit). The more oil glands present in the plant, the cheaper the oil, and vice versa. For instance, 100 kilograms of lavender yields almost 3 litres of essential oil, whereas 1000 kilograms of rose petals yields only half a litre.

Each essential oil is a complex synergistic mix of various organic chemicals and represents the dynamic healing properties of the plant. It is believed to contain its life force, having certain therapeutic or balancing effects. Because of this synergy, essential oils do not disturb the body's natural balance, or homeostasis; if one component has a strong effect another component acts as a balancer, or quencher, therefore making essential oils highly versatile and safe in healing practice. Essential oils are highly concentrated substances and rarely used neat, though neat lavender essence is sometimes used in first aid and as an antiseptic.

In aromatherapy, inhalation, application and baths are the principal methods used to encourage essential oils to enter the body. Because essential oils are highly volatile, evaporating readily on exposure to air, and when inhaled may enter the body via the olfactory system, when diluted and applied externally, essential oil molecules may permeate the skin. Bath treatments enable you to both inhale and absorb the oils. Once within your system, essential oils will work to re-establish harmony and revitalise those systems or organs where there is a malfunction or lack of balance.

Essential oils also act on the central nervous system. Some will relax (chamomile, lavender, rose otto); others will stimulate (rosemary, jasmine, black pepper, eucalyptus). A few have the ability to 'normalise', for example, hyssop can raise low blood pressure and lower high blood pressure. Likewise, bergamot and geranium can either sedate or stimulate according to individual needs. Some researchers have indicated that essential oils can increase atmospheric oxygen and provide negative ions, inhibiting bacterial growth, thereby rendering them antibacterial and anti-infectious.

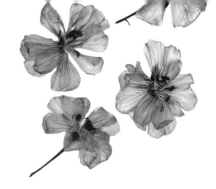

HOW ESSENTIAL OILS WORK

Essential oils are used as a gentle approach to healthcare, to aid skincare, soothe and promote relaxation and simply to seduce us with the world of fragrant treasures. These oils work on us at physical, physiological and psychological levels. At a psychological level they work through inhalation, while skin application helps at the physical and physiological level. Essential oils are also beneficial at the subtle level for cleansing the aura and chakras; along with cleansing the environment from negative energies, this has been the reason for their use in spiritual practices.

PSYCHOLOGICAL EFFECT

The part of the brain that identifies aromas is called the limbic section, or the central part of the brain; it is also responsible for our memory and emotions. When inhaled, essential oil molecules are taken directly to the olfactory system, which is a patch of cells located on the roof of our nose. These cells have minute, hair-like protrusions called cilia which register and transmit information about the aromas to our brain via the olfactory nerve, which is directly connected to the brain. When electrochemical messages about the odour are forwarded to the limbic section of the brain, it triggers the release of neurotransmitters, which may result in relaxing, uplifting, sedative or euphoric effects on our body through hormones released by our pituitary gland. The balancing effect essential oils can have on the mind lends an added dimension to their use in healing stress-related/psychosomatic disorders. All essential oils help to balance emotions to some degree.

PHYSICAL/PHYSIOLOGICAL EFFECTS

When dissolved in a carrier oil and rubbed into the skin or when dispersed in water used for a bath, tiny essential oil molecules, being volatile in nature, readily permeate the skin via the skin pores and hair follicles.

They reach the body's circulatory system through the lymphatic vessels. Once in the bloodstream they are transported around the body and are filtered through to the bodily fluids, passing their therapeutic benefits to the entire body. Since essential oils with inherent therapeutic properties are able to keep infection at bay, they boost the entire functioning of the immune system.

EFFECT OF ESSENTIAL OILS ON BIOFREQUENCY

For years, research has been conducted on the use of electrical energy to reverse disease. Scientists in the field of natural and energy healing have believed there has to be a more natural way to increase the body's electrical frequency. This led to the research into and subsequent discovery of electrical frequencies in essential oils.

Every living thing has energy which can be measured in terms of electrical frequency. Frequency is a measurable rate of electrical energy that is constant between any two points. Considerable research has been done; Robert O Becker, MD, documented the electrical frequency of the human body in his book called *The Body Electric*. Bruce Tainio of Tainio Technology in Cheney, Washington, developed a way to measure the biofrequency of humans and foods using biofrequency monitors to determine the relationship between frequency and disease. Measuring in megahertz, it was found that a healthy body typically has a frequency ranging from 62 to 78 megahertz (MHz), while the process of disease sets in at 58 MHz. This energy level gets disturbed even by a single negative thought. In studies it was observed that negative thoughts lowered the measured frequency of a person up to 12 MHz and positive thoughts raised the measured frequency by 10 MHz. It was also found that prayer and meditation increased the measured frequency levels by 15 MHz. This gives credence to the idea that prolonged levels of stress, anxiety, depression, etc., result in lowering the body's energy as well as immunity levels, allowing disease to set in, as the case is in all psychosomatic disorders.

It was also observed in those studies that processed food had a zero to minimal MHz frequency, fresh produce measured up to 15 MHz, dried herbs from 12–22 MHz and fresh herbs from 20–27 MHz. Essential oils have been found to have the highest frequency of natural substances, starting at 52 MHz and going as high as 320 MHz, the frequency of rose oil. In this sense, the chemistry and frequencies of essential oils have the ability to help us maintain optimal health frequency providing an environment where microbes cannot live.

When essential oils were diffused it was observed that patients felt better emotionally, within seconds of exposure to the oils, and inhalation of the same resulted in them feeling calmer and less anxious. It is fascinating to see the way the oils work on the body; certain oils acted within seconds while others acted in 1–3 minutes; when oil was applied to the feet it could travel to the head and take effect within a minute. With such positive results, more and more studies are being initiated in this field.

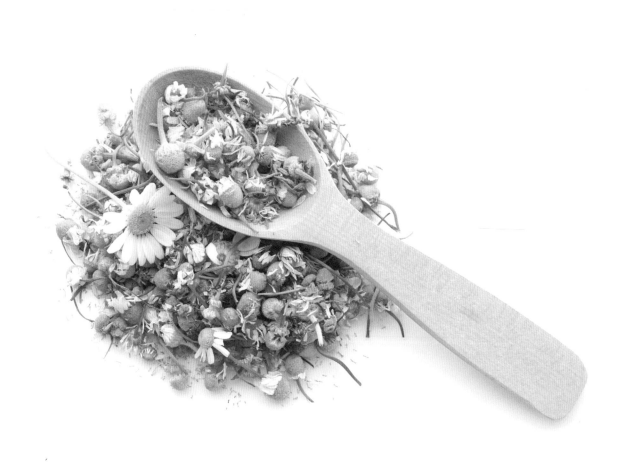

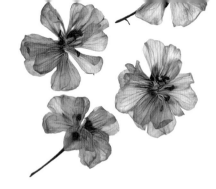

AROMA CHEMISTRY

The way plants make essential oils gives some insight into their complexity. The primary and secondary metabolism of the plants has been the subject of study for organic- and biochemists. The chemical components of an essential oil are produced during the second stage of biosynthesis and thus are secondary metabolites. (Secondary metabolites are those chemical compounds in organisms that are not directly involved in the normal growth, development or reproduction of an organism.)

A distilled essential oil is a mixture of various organic chemicals, some of which are present as natural constituents of the oil at the time of distillation, others are formed during processing by the hydrolysis of glycosides, while a few are formed by partial decomposition of delicate natural components.

The chemistry of essential oils is complex. The components of the essential oils can broadly be classified as terpenes, esters, aldehydes, ketones, alcohols, phenols and oxides. Since essential oils are composed of a wide range of different chemicals, they all have different therapeutic effects and affect the body in different ways. This explains why a single essential oil can have a wide range of therapeutic properties. Lavender, for example, balances the central nervous system and is also a wonderful skin-healing agent for problems such as athlete's foot, bedsores, acne and eczema. The essential oil can also be used in the bath or blended into a massage oil for a relaxing or therapeutic massage to relieve conditions like muscular pain and rheumatism, and much more. It is interesting to note that resins such as frankincense and myrrh containing resin alcohols have a similar chemical structure to human steroids (the male and female hormones). Whether resin alcohols exert a hormone-stimulating effect on humans has not been officially proven. Much more research into this area is needed before we dare jump to any firm conclusions.

The gas chromatograph can separate out the main components of essential oils by looking at the 'chemical fingerprint' produced. However, the pattern of the living essence is complex, well beyond the chemist's ability to replicate the exact aroma by mixing together the various chemical components. Something is always missing in the 'nature identical' version. Following are the main components and therapeutic effects of the isolated constituents found in essential oils.

Terpenes make up the largest single group of compounds in essential oils. Normally their name ends in '-ene'. Terpenes are made up of a chain of 5 carbon atoms, one of them having a double bond, known as an isoprene unit. Depending on the number of isoprene units in a terpenic compound, it can be classified as monoterpene, sesquiterpene or diterpene.

Monoterpenes are composed of two isoprene units. This is the basic terpene, making up the largest group of terpenes. They are light molecules, hence evaporate quickly when exposed to air, thus represent themselves in top notes. Since the isoprenes making the terpenes have double bonds, they are prone to oxidation, therefore they are photosensitive. Essential oils rich in terpenes have a short shelf life.

Common monoterpenes include limonene (an antiviral agent found in 90 per cent of citrus oils), pinene (an antiseptic found in high concentrations in pine and turpentine oils), camphene and myrcene. They are mild antiseptics and have an uplifting and stimulating effect on the nervous system.

Sesquiterpenes are composed of three isoprene units, making them slightly heavier and less volatile. They have a stronger odour and anti-inflammatory and bactericidal properties. Common examples are chamazulene (German chamomile), bisabolene (black pepper) and caryophyllene (ylang ylang).

Diterpenes are heavy molecules made up of four isoprene units. They are not common as they tend to react with hydroxyl groups to form terpenic alcohols. This process in clary sage produces sclareol, a component known for its hormone-balancing effect.

Alcohols Terpenic alcohols, ending in '-ol', are found in many essential oils. They are the result of the reaction of terpenes with hydroxyl groups (OH). Monoterpenic alcohols are good antiseptics with some antibacterial and antifungal properties. Some alcohols are uplifting; others, such as linalool, have a sedative effect, while isoborneol inhibits the herpes virus (Armaka et al 1999). Diterpenic alcohols such as sclareol have a hormone regulating effect.

Essential oils having a higher percentage of monoterpenic alcohols are safe to be used on skin, even undiluted. Some of the most common terpene alcohols include linalool (found in lavender), citronellol (rose and geranium) and geraniol (geranium and palmarosa). These substances tend to give good antiseptic and antiviral properties, as well as uplifting qualities to essential oils.

Esters The most widespread group found in plant essences. Ending in '-ate', esters are combination of an acid with an alcohol, for example linalylic acid combined with alcohol produces linalyl acetate, found in clary sage and lavender. Geranyl acetate is found in geranium and sweet marjoram. Esters are fungicidal, antispasmodic and sedative, usually with a fruity aroma.

Aldehydes are found notably in lemon-scented essences ending in '-al', such as citral in lemongrass and citronella, as well as cinnamic aldehyde in cinnamon oil. They are strong chemicals which can sensitise the skin and should therefore be used with caution. Aldehydes generally have antidepressant and uplifting qualities.

Ketones The ketones found in pennyroyal, tansy, sage and wormwood are toxic, which is why these essences are best avoided by the layperson. Ending in 'one' (such as thujone in wormwood), they are aromatic chemicals with a strong aroma. However, not all ketones are dangerous. Non-toxic ketones include jasmone, found in jasmine, and fenchone in sweet fennel. Ketones ease congestion and aid the flow of mucus, which is why plants and essences containing these substances are helpful for upper respiratory complaints.

Phenols are bactericidal with a strong and stimulating effect on the central nervous system. They are aromatic group alcohols and also end in '-ol'. However, they are stronger chemicals and can also be skin irritants, especially if isolated from the whole essential oil and used as single 'active principle'. Common phenols such as eugenol in clove oil and thymol in thyme oil are potentially harmful so it is best to avoid using these essences, at least for skin use. Clove essence, for instance, can be safely used in room perfumes.

Oxides are found in a wide range of essences, especially those of camphoraceous nature such as eucalyptus oil, which contains an oxide called 1–8 cineole or eucalyptol, and has an expectorant effect.

THE THERAPEUTIC EFFECTS OF ESSENTIAL OIL COMPONENTS

	Acids	Alcohols (mono)	Alcohols (sesqui)	Aldehydes	Coumarins	Esters	Esters (phenolic)	Ketones	Lactones	Oxides	Phenols	Terpenes (mono)	Terpenes (sesqui)
Abortifacient								x					
Analgesic								x			x	x	x
Air antiseptic											x		
Antiseptic				x							x		x
Anticoagulant					x			x					
Anti-fungal		x		x		x		x					
Ant-infectious		x		x			x				x		
Anti-infammatory	x			x		x	x	x					x
Anti-spasmodic						x	x				x		x
Antiviral		x		x							x	x	
Bactericidal		x									x	x	x
Balancing					x								
Cicatrisant						x		x			x		
Decongestant (circulatory)			x										
Digestive								x			x		
Diuretic											x		
Expectorant								x		x	x	x	
Hepatic		x	x										
Hypotensive		x	x	x									x
Immune system balancer		x											
Immunostimulant										x			
Lipolytic								x					
Mucolytic								x	x	x	x		
Neurotoxic								x					
Phototoxic					x								
Relaxant				x	x	x	x	x				x	
Sedative				x			x	x			x		
Skin irritant				x						x	x	x	
Skin sensitising				x					x				
Stimulant		x						x				x	
Temperature reducing			x	x						x			
Tonic, nerve (uplifting)		x	x			x	x	x			x		
Tonic (general)		x	x	x									
Vasoconstrictive		x											
Warming		x									x		

Lactones are present in all expressed oils. The percentage may be low but they play an important role as they are expectorant and mucolytic, although some lactones have a neurotoxic effect as ketones.

Coumarins are a type or subgroup like lactones. They may be present in an oil in a small quantity and have antispasmodic effect. A certain group of coumarins present in citrus peels, such as bergaptine in bergamot (*Citrus bergamia*), and also found in angelica root, react in the presence of ultraviolet light, so can cause phototoxicity.

Ethers are responsible for some of the hallucinogenic properties of certain essential oils when taken orally.

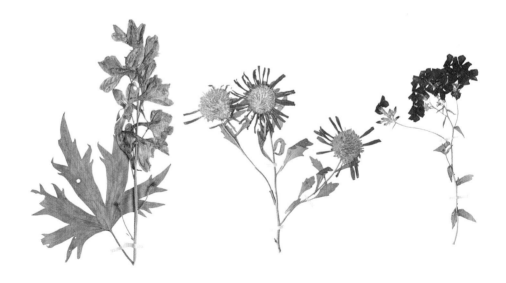

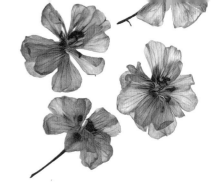

VOLATILITY OF ESSENTIAL OILS

The volatility of an essential oil is the rate of evaporation of its components.

We can smell the aroma of certain essential oils as soon as we open the bottle, while in other cases we need to bring a container close to our nose to get a whiff. This is because essential oils evaporate at different rates depending on their composition. The organic chemicals that make up an essential oil can be light or heavy. An essential oil composed of lighter chemicals evaporates quickly and instantly hits our nose; these are called 'top note' oils. For example, monoterpenes, monoterpenols, ketones, phenols, aldehydes and oxides show themselves in 'top notes', hence oils with a higher percentage of these components have a strong aroma. When an oil has mid-size chemicals, comparatively slower to evaporate, they show themselves in 'middle notes', including sesquiterpenes, sesquiterpenols, esters and alcohols. The heavy components, including diterpenes, diterpenols and wax esters, take longer to evaporate and are called 'base notes'. These components act as natural fixatives as they help to hold the lighter components. Base note oils are also good moisturisers as they help bind moisture to the skin.

All fragrances, whether natural or synthetic, can be classified as top, middle and bottom notes. In a perfume or essential oil (a single oil may contain more than one note), the top note is the initial aroma we smell, followed by middle notes, which are slightly different but longer lasting, making up the body of the perfume, then what you smell when the perfume has almost evaporated are the bottom or base notes.

The art of blending involves creating a balance of top, middle and bottom note oils or components. Normally we use a combination of three to five essential oils, as they are synergists (i.e. they increase the therapeutic effect of other essential oils and control the side effects). Whether mixing oils for vaporisation, a bath or as a perfume, we need to be aware of the aroma effect as well as the therapeutic effect of the oil.

TOP NOTES

Aromas classified as top notes are highly uplifting, stimulating the mind and relieving depression. They are cleansing and invigorating, help clear congestion and colds, and also help in respiratory conditions. Typical top note oils include citrus, leafy, camphoraceous and minty aromas; for example, lemon, lime, bergamot orange, grapefruit, lemongrass, melissa, peppermint, spearmint, basil, rosemary, eucalyptus and jasmine.

MIDDLE NOTES

Most of the middle note oils are extracted from flowers, berries, herbs and spices. They are mostly relaxing and healing, help reduce hypertension, and are also good for PMS and related symptoms. Examples include lavender, geranium, chamomiles, clary sage, ylang ylang, juniper berry, marjoram, clove, nutmeg, black pepper and ginger.

BOTTOM/BASE NOTES

Base note oils are soothing, relaxing sedatives, lingering and help restore emotional balance. Extracted from roots, wood, stems, bark and resins, they are used as fixatives and moisturisers. Examples include vetiver, patchouli, sandalwood, cedarwood, myrrh, benzoin, jatamansi and valerian root oil.

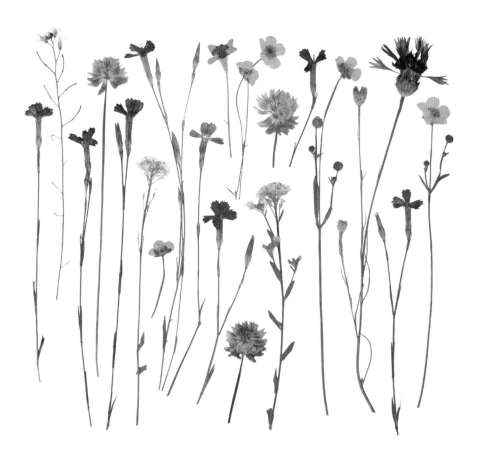

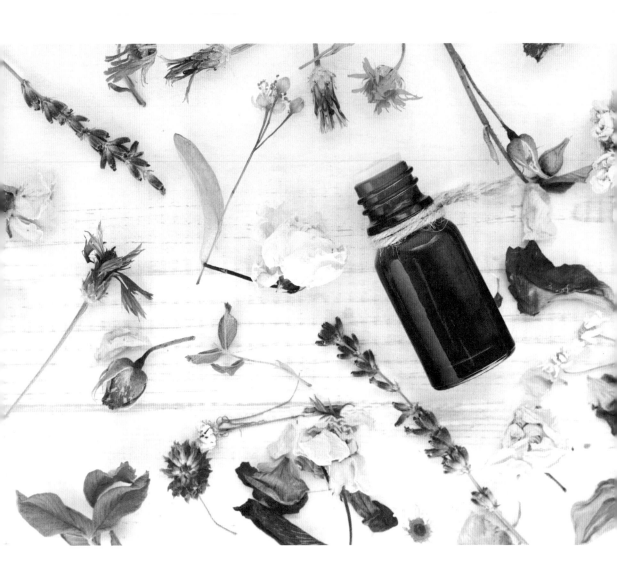

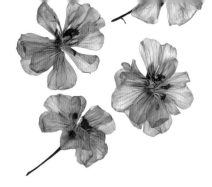

EXTRACTION METHODS

The basic principles for extracting essential oils from plants remain the same as those of hundreds of years ago, although tremendous advances have been made in the techniques used and the methods employed. An oil extractor's objective is to extract essential oil in the most natural form. Distillation is, and no doubt will continue to be, the most important of these.

Essential oils are contained in the glands, veins, sacs and glandular hairs of aromatic plants. Flowers, leaves and non-fibrous parts need little if any preparation prior to distillation. Tough stalks, woody parts, roots, seeds and fruits, however, need to be comminuted (cut up, disintegrated or crushed – wood is grated) in order to rupture the cell walls, allowing the easy escape of the volatile oil.

During distillation, only very tiny molecules can evaporate, so they are the only ones which leave the plant. These extremely small molecules make up an essential oil. Oils containing more of the smallest molecules are most volatile, the 'top notes' of the perfumery world; those containing more of the heaviest and least volatile of tiny molecules are 'base notes'.

STEAM DISTILLATION

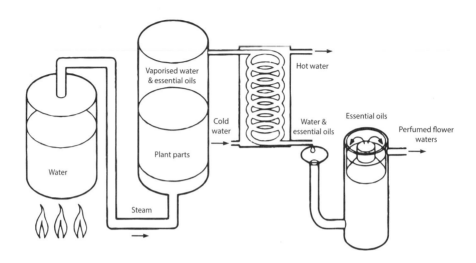

Distillation is still considered to be one of the most economical methods of extracting essential oils from plant materials. Some plants need to be distilled immediately after they have been harvested. For example, if melissa is left even for a few hours, the essential oil is lost; hence the yield from melissa is very low. However, some plants, such as lavender, are left a few days so that surplus water in the plant can dry out (this slightly affects the yield). Some, like black pepper seeds, clary sage and peppermint, can be totally dried before distilling without losing any essential oil. There is an art to distillation and, especially for low-yield plants, much skill is needed. The aim of the distiller is to achieve an oil as close as possible to the oil as it exists in the plant.

When plants are heated by steam in a still, the essential oils present in the plant material are freed, evaporating into the steam. These tiny molecules are carried along a pipe together with the steam and as they get further away from the heat source they begin to cool. To hasten this process, the pipe passes through a large vat of cold water where steam condenses back into liquid form. As the density of essential oil differs from that of water, it either floats on the top or sinks to the bottom (mostly the former) where it can be drawn off. The result is pure, genuine, whole and natural essential oil – an aromatherapist's dream.

CARBON DIOXIDE EXTRACTION

This method of extracting essential oils was introduced at the beginning of the 1980s and utilises compressed carbon dioxide (CO_2). The technology calls for expensive and complicated equipment which utilises CO_2 at very high pressure and extremely low temperature. With this method, more top notes, fewer terpenes, a higher proportion of esters plus larger molecules can be obtained. The resultant oil is said to be better and more like the essential oil in the plant, as many terpenes seem to form during the distillation process, which also breaks down some of the acetates (esters) in the plant material.

CO_2-extracted essential oils are pure and stable, colourless and have no residue of CO_2 left in them – thus they are excellent therapeutically, although this needs to be verified for each oil, given their different compositions.

This method is not suitable for all oils; there are still a few practical difficulties to overcome (for example, sometimes an emulsion is produced).

HYDRO DIFFUSION OR PERCOLATION

Percolation is a more recent method than CO_2 extraction. Most of the resultant oils have an aroma closer to that of the plant, better than a distilled oil. The equipment, unlike that for CO_2 extraction, is very simple and the process quicker than distillation, the plant being in contact with the steam for a much shorter time, thus truer to nature.

This process works like a coffee percolator. The steam passes through the plant material from top to bottom of the container, which has a grid to hold the plant material. The oil and condensed steam is collected in a vessel in the same way as distillation. The colour of the oils is much richer than that of distilled oils and time and tests alone will reveal their true value in aromatherapy.

EXPRESSION

This method of extraction is used exclusively with citrus fruits, where the essential oil, located in little sacs just under the surface of the rind, simply needs to be pressed out.

Expression is usually carried out by a factory producing fruit juice, thus maximising the profit from the whole fruit. Expressed oil is taken directly from the fresh peel without heat. It is recommended that citrus oils for therapeutic use be obtained from organically or naturally grown produce.

Cold-pressed citrus oils are preferable as they are known to be of exactly the same composition as the plant itself. In many juice/essential oil factories, the peel is steam distilled after expression, which releases even more oil (though of a poorer quality).

In the past, the oil was extracted by hand (and collected in sponges), however, the size of the industry today necessitates expression by machinery and the process is known as 'scarification'. With expression, both volatile and large molecules such as waxes and other substances are contained in the finished product, while by distillation only tiny molecules can be collected.

The shelf life of expressed oils is shorter than that of distilled oils. They should be stored in a cool, dark place (many people choose the refrigerator).

SOLVENT EXTRACTION

Resinoids, concretes and absolutes are obtained by solvent extraction and not classed as essential oils. They are highly concentrated perfume materials, containing those plant molecules that are soluble in the solvents used to extract them.

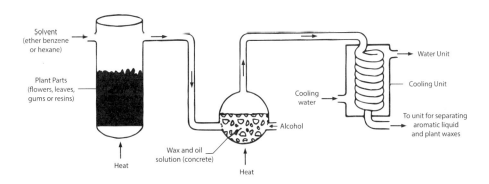

Resinoid

Resins are the solid or semi-solid substances exuded from the bark of trees and shrubs when wounded (cut, as in a rubber tree). The gum-like substance is produced pathologically, solely as a result of the incision, and hardens on exposure to air. Various solvents can be used to extract the aromatic molecules from resin, the most frequently used being hydrocarbons (for example, benzene or hexane) or alcohols, each extracting different molecules. The solvents are filtered off and afterward removed by distillation to leave either resinoids (from hydrocarbon solvents) or absolute resins (from alcohol solvents). Commonly used absolutes from resins and their extracts in aromatherapy are frankincense, benzoin, myrrh, elemi and galbanum.

Concretes

As for resinoids, the extraction of Solventcretes also uses hydrocarbons as a solvent. Concretes, however, are extracted from plant material (leaves, flowers, roots, etc.). Most concretes are solid, waxlike substances and much used in food flavourings.

Absolutes

An absolute is prepared from a concrete by adding an alcohol to extract the aromatic (alcohol-soluble) molecules. The alcohol is then evaporated off gently under vacuum, leaving the absolute, a thick, coloured liquid. The total process is much more complicated.

Absolutes and resins always retain a small percentage of the solvents used in their production, so not preferred for aromatherapy work, but they are much used in the perfumery world. Some solvents may cause substance sensitivity on certain skins, depending on the quality and quantity of the retained solvent. Jasmine absolute, a favourite aroma for many people and possibly the most important fragrance to the perfume industry (there is no essential oil of jasmine available), is extremely vulnerable to adulteration and available at a wide range of prices reflecting the quality.

Enfleurage

Pomades were obtained from the enfleurage process used long ago (replaced by concretes), when petals or leaves were laid on trays of animal fat for many days, being replaced regularly until the fat being used as a solvent was saturated with the plant extracts.

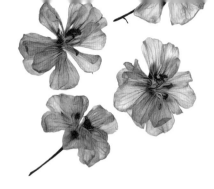

QUALITY CONTROL OF ESSENTIAL OILS

In the practice of aromatherapy, the quality of essential oils plays a very important role. These days, people try to cash in on the popularity of aromatherapy by dishing out all sorts of essential oils, from synthetic/reconstituted or 'nature identical' to adulterated. We have to be careful about the quality of the essential oils we use for therapy purposes or the desired result will not be obtained.

Traditionally, the purpose of quality control has been to make sure that substandard products do not reach the customer. It is very important to check the quality of essential oils as optimum quality is paramount not only in order to get best results but also to avoid possible harmful side effects. Another bonus is that less high-quality essential oil is needed in order to be effective, so buying cheaper oils is a false economy.

The quality of essential oils can be tested by non-analytical physical tests or analytical tests.

NON-ANALYTICAL PHYSICAL TESTS

Non-analytical physical tests give information on certain properties of essential oils, though not on their composition.

Appearance: The appearance of an essential oil is no criterion of good quality, but may warn of poor quality. Most distilled oils of high quality are either transparent or slightly hazy. A definitely hazy or cloudy essential oil is always of questionable quality. Absolutes frequently present a hazy, translucent or even opaque appearance. Expressed citrus oils are always coloured and show natural colour variations due to difference in the pigmentation in the outer rind of the fruit.

Viscosity: This refers to the thickness of a liquid or, more scientifically, to its resistance to flow, commonly seen in high-viscosity liquids such as glycerine. Water, conversely, is a mobile liquid, one of low viscosity. All expressed and most distilled oils used in aromatherapy are mobile liquids, while a few like sandalwood, vetiver and jatamansi are viscous. Few essential oils, like orris oil, for example are solid at room temperature.

Specific gravity: The specific gravity of a solid or liquid is a measure of how much heavier or lighter a given volume of the substance is than the same volume of pure water, measured at a standard temperature. Measurement of specific gravity is usually made at 20 degrees Celsius. The specific gravity of water is 1. Most essential oils are lighter than water so have a specific gravity of less than 1, but a few, for example clove oil, are heavier and collect beneath the distillation water during extraction.

Today, specific gravity is measured by means of an electronic specific gravity meter which gives the result and temperature of the sample on a small LCD display screen.

Refractive index: When you lower a needle into a bowl of water at an angle of about 60 degrees to the horizontal, the needle appears to bend towards the surface as it enters the water and unbend as it is withdrawn. This optical effect is called 'refraction', caused by the reduction of speed of light when passing from a less dense medium (in this case air) into a denser medium (water). The refraction of a ray of light passing from air into a transparent liquid or solid medium is expressed numerically as the refractive index of the denser medium, for example, an essential oil, with respect to the air.

As in the case of specific gravity, a specification of refractive index is expressed as upper and lower limits between which, at the given temperature, the refractive index of the test sample should lie.

The property of refraction of light can be very responsive to small changes of composition, so for an essential oil, a value for refractive index that is greater or lesser than the limits of the specified range is regarded as an early warning of the possibility of poor quality, to the extent of adulteration.

Refractive index is measured with a refractometer, using a thin film of test sample mounted on a temperature-controlled stage, similar to the stage of a microscope. A standard light source gives a visual field, viewed through one of the two eyepieces, consisting of adjacent semicircles of coloured light. The field is adjusted by the operator to show an even distribution of colour, whereupon the refractive index of the sample is obtained on a scale, visible through the other eyepiece. Electronic refractometers give direct readings of refractive index free from human observational error.

Examples of the refractive indices of essential oils:

Bergamot oil: 1.464 to 1.467
Clove bud oil: 1.528 to 1.537
Lavender oil: 1.459 to 1.464
Lemongrass oil 1.483 to 1.489
Rosemary oil: 1.464 to 1.476
Sandalwood oil: 1.500 to 1.510

Optical rotation: Light waves are analogous to the waves produced in a long length of rope secured at one end when the opposite end is moved energetically up and down; they are traverse waves, propagated in a plane perpendicular to the surface to which rope is secured. A polarised lens of the kind used for sunglasses is used, since this material absorbs all rays of light passing through it, except those travelling in a particular plane called the plane of polarisation. Rays emerging from such a filter are plane-polarised, meaning that all of them travel in parallel planes.

Optical rotation is measured with a polariscope. A polariscope tube (a 10-centimetre-long horizontal glass tube fitted with plane glass ends) is filled with the liquid under examination. To measure optical rotation of essential oils, the temperature of the tube and contents are adjusted to a level between 15 and 20 degrees Celsius and the tube is then placed horizontally in the polariscope. A beam of plane-polarised light of sodium wavelength is passed through the liquid and viewed at the opposite end through an eyepiece fitted with a second polarising lens secured to a circular scale marked in angular degrees. The scale is rotated until the two halves of an illuminated field, as viewed through the eyepiece, are equally illuminated, whereupon a reading is taken from the scale.

If the liquid in the polariscope tube is optically inactive (for example, water), the scale of reading will be zero. Indeed, the zero reading of the instrument can be checked in this way if necessary before a measurement is made. If the liquid is optically active, it will twist the plane-polarised light waves emerging from the first polarising lens (the polariser) clockwise or anticlockwise as they pass through it. Hence to obtain a uniformly illuminated viewing field, the second polarising lens (the analyser) must be rotated by moving the circular scale to which it is attached. The angle of optical rotation is then obtained from the scale reading.

Liquids which rotate the plane of the polarised light to the right (clockwise) are said to be dextrorotatory, and the names of the organic compounds of this nature are prefixed as d-, for example d-limonene. Liquids which rotate the plane of polarised light to the left (anticlockwise) are laevorotatory. The names of laevorotatory compounds are prefixed l-, such as l-limonene. The explanation of optical activity throws light, so as to speak, on the composition of essential oils, since optical activity is caused by a particular feature of molecular structure in which an atom, particularly a carbon atom, is bonded to four different atoms or group of atoms.

The optical rotation of an essential oil is a summation of the optical rotations of its constituents in relation to their proportions in the oil. These proportions affect the therapeutic properties of the oil. Variations of these proportions can cause variations of the optical rotation of the oil, so measurement of optical rotation is an important aid to the detection of adulteration. For example, when a deficiency of a major, optically active constituent has been corrected by the addition of the corresponding, non-stereospecific synthetic chemical, since the optical activity of the aroma chemical will be different from the natural component, adulteration of the oil with aroma chemical will therefore alter the value of its optical rotation.

ANALYTICAL CHEMICAL TESTS

Analytical chemistry may be defined as the science and art of determining the composition of material in terms of the elements or compounds contained.

There are two basic kinds of analytical tests: **qualitative**, giving information on what is present in a substance, and **quantitative**, giving information on how much constituent of a mixture or element is present in a compound.

Qualitative tests

From the results of qualitative tests on an essential oil, the identity of one or more of its different constituents may be ascertained after separation from the oil.

Acid value: With advancing age, the content of free acid in many essential oils tends to increase. This increase results mainly from the oxidation of aldehydes and hydrolysis of esters to form equivalent quantities of organic acids, the stronger of which can catalyse the further hydrolysis of esters.

The measurement of the acid content of an essential oil, expressed as 'acid value', and comparison of the result with the acid value quoted as the maximum acceptable in the specification for the oil, gives an indication of the condition and age of the product and by inference its likely rate of deterioration – a guide to whether the oil is usable or not. In the absence of deterioration, the proportion of free acid to be found in most essential oils is very small.

Determination of esters: Some essential oils, for example lavender, are valued for their content of natural esters (linalyl acetate and other esters in the case of lavender). An ester value lower than that prescribed in the specification is a certain indication of poor quality.

Quantitative tests

Quantitative information about the individual components of an essential oil is usually obtained by the technique of gas-liquid chromatography. However, chemical tests are also used to evaluate the quality of all constituents of a particular chemical class present in an oil, for example, the total percentage of esters calculated as linalyl acetate, present in lavender oil.

Gas-liquid chromatography (GLC): 'Chromatography' is basically the separation of components present in a chemical mixture. Chromatography may be regarded as an analytical technique employed for the purification and separation of organic and inorganic substances. There are several different chromatographic techniques.

Gas-liquid chromatography, also called capillary GLC, is used in perfumery and essential oils analysis for its sensitivity, separating power and reproducibility of results. The column takes the form of a narrow silica tube of less than 1 millimetre internal diameter chromatrograph and from 30 to 100 m in length, which is wound into a coil on a former and coated on the inside with a very thin film of a non-volatile substance. The column is secured within a temperature-regulated, thermostatically controlled oven, the temperature of which can be computer-programmed to increase, over a period of about 30 minutes, from room temperature to above 300 degrees Celsius. This is important to ensure that all constituents, from the least to most volatile, are vaporised slowly.

One end of the column is attached to a metal block (the injection block) with a fine hole, from which one minute drop of an essential oil is injected for analysis. The block is preheated to ensure that the essential oil evaporates as soon as it is injected. At the point of evaporation there is a connection to a cylinder of nitrogen gas, which is chemically inert and acts as a carrier, to carry the vapours of the sample through the column. The carrier gas is basically the 'moving phase' in GLC analysis.

At the opposite end of the column is a device called the detector, which is connected to a pen recorder. The detector responds quantitatively to the presence of the truly minute amount of the vapours of the constituents separated by the column. The variations in this current, once amplified, are converted into exactly proportional movements of the pen recorder, in which the pen is arranged to draw a line on a slowly moving sheet of paper. The pen draws a peak on the paper as a permanent record of its presence and proportions in the sample. The electrical signals (changes of current) produced by the detector are also fed into a dedicated computer known as the integrator, which, on completion of analysis, prints out sets of figures from which the constituents of the sample can be identified and their true proportions calculated.

For the results of different GLC analyses to be comparable, the conditions of column parameters (length, diameter, composition and thickness of the stationary phase, etc.) and temperature, temperature programming, nature and flow of carrier gas, all have to be standardised and kept the same from one analysis to the next.

The purpose of the routine evaluation of a fresh supply of essential oil received is to compare the chromatograph with the corresponding, standard samples which are of known composition and which conform in each case to the quality required.

Infrared spectrophotometry (IRS): The technique of infrared spectrophotometry involves measuring of the energy of different parts of the spectrum of infrared radiation. Applied to an essential oil, IRS gives an overall picture, or fingerprint, of the composition of the oil. The IR spectrograph is very sensitive to small differences of composition, and so is a most useful aid to the comparison of test and standard samples of essential oils, and to the detection of adulteration. The technique also has the advantage of being able to detect and record the presence of non-volatile as well as volatile constituents of essential oils, and of requiring only a few minutes for the completion of a spectrum.

Mass spectrometry: This analytical technique is a powerful aid to the elucidation of the composition and structure of molecules of chemically pure organic compounds. For the purpose of the elucidation of the molecular structure of constituents of essential oils, a pure constituent separated by GLC and represented by a single peak on a chromatograph is transferred directly to a mass spectrometer.

Concepts of purity

The word 'pure' refers to a product free from contamination or adulteration. In the case of essential oils, there are two concepts of purity: odour purity and chemical purity.

Odour purity may be defined as the extent to which the odour profile matches the odour profile of a standard sample of the same product and grade when both are allowed to evaporate on smelling strips to final dry out under the same conditions at the same time. Careful odour evaluation at intervals during evaporation under standard conditions and in comparison with a standard sample is very important in essential oils and the only test available to aromatherapists besides visual inspection.

Chemical purity can be checked in chemicals that have identical atoms or molecules, however, the concept only applies to single elements or compounds. An essential oil, being a mixture of organic compounds, cannot be chemically pure, even though it may be of high odour purity and 'pure' in the sense of being free from contamination. The chemical composition and odour profile of an essential oil together provide the information from which its purity can be ascertained, in comparison with a standard sample.

FACTORS DETERMINING THE QUALITY

The composition and quality of essential oils is determined by the following factors:

1. Genotype of the plant source: The genetic constitution of the plant determines the composition of the proteins forming the living matter, or protoplasm, of the plant. These proteins include the enzymes, which control the metabolism of the plant. In aromatic plants, essential oils are formed in oil glands or cells, their composition being determined by the enzyme-controlled reaction pathways by which their constituents are synthesised.

2. Conditions of growth and development of the plant: These are a major factor affecting the quality of essential oil. A green plant obtains the chemical elements that it requires for growth and development to maturity from the surrounding atmosphere and from the soil by which it is supported. Deficiencies of any of the ions required by a plant causes poor growth and yellowing of leaves and, in aromatic plants, poor yield of inferior quality essential oils. Atmospheric pollution can damage or destroy plant life, as can contaminated soil.

3. Harvesting and processing of aromatic plant material is another important factor determining whether a high yield of good quality essential oil is obtained. The source material must be harvested at the time when its oil content is at its maximum, using a technique that excludes extraneous matter, such as weeds. Care with processing is vital to ensure completion of the extraction process in the shortest possible time but under conditions of temperature and pressure that will not cause any part of the charge in the still to suffer damaging thermal stress.

4. Effect of moisture on essential oils is an important factor to be taken care of before final packing, as essential oils produced by expression or distillation frequently contain proportions of dissolved water. Some

oils are comparatively more stable in the presence of moisture while others (such as citrus plant oils) are not.

5. **Storage conditions:** In general, essential oils should be stored under the following conditions:

- In a cool place, at an even temperature
- Protected from light
- Under nitrogen
- In non-plastic containers, the material of which will not in any way alter their composition.

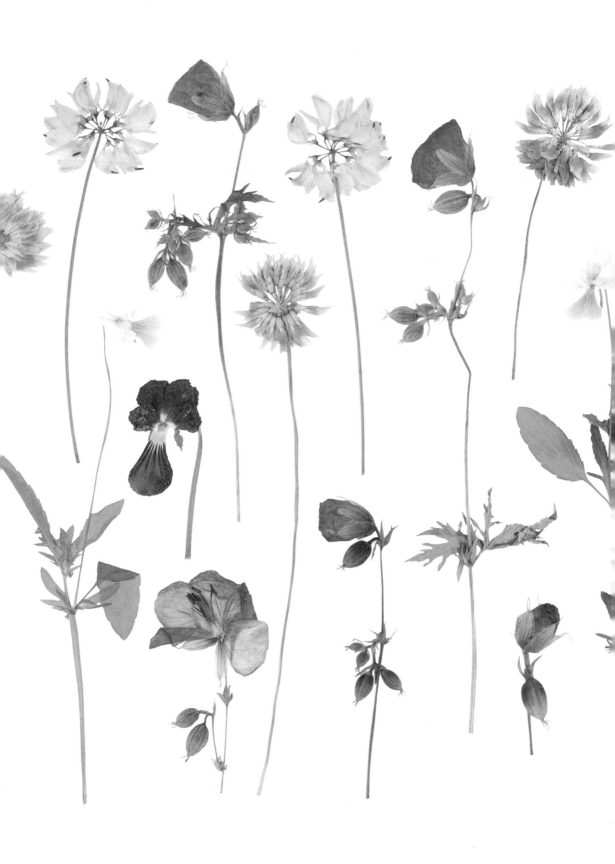

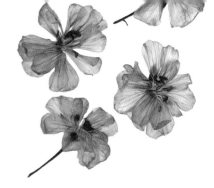

PLANT FAMILIES

When aromatherapy was first introduced, essential oils were referred to by their common plant name. However, this can be confusing, as different plants may have the same common name. For example, marjoram (*Origanum majorana*) may be confused with oregano (*O. vulgare*), which is sometimes also referred to as 'marjoram'. They are both in the genus *Origanum* and their oils may contain common factors, yet they have a different aroma as well as different therapeutic effects on the human system. One needs to know which essential oil from which species is needed for which purpose.

Other plants with the same common name may not even be related, sharing neither the same genus nor species. For example, a European aromatherapist may refer to 'cypress', meaning *Cupressus sempervirens*, while in India 'cypress' may refer to nagarmotha or cypriol (*Cyperus scariosus*).

As knowledge on the subject has deepened, the necessity of using the Latin names has become more apparent; it is now vital for plant oils to be precisely identified. A plant may have many common names but only one specific two-part Latin name.

Carl Linnaeus (1707–1778) formalised binomial nomenclature, the modern system of naming organisms. Every plant name is composed of two Latin names. The first name represents its genus (a particular family group) and the second is the name of its species (representing plants having similar properties, which may or may not be from same geographical region). The classification of plants (and other organisms) is called taxonomy, which categorises them into division, class, order, family, genus and species. This process takes into account a number of factors: geographical; climatic; type of plant; type of stem; number, shape and position of leaves on the stem; the shape and position of flowers; number and shape of petals; whether the plant is hairy, prickly or smooth, and so on.

If an essential oil is labelled and known only by its common name, not only can the incorrect use of a powerful, possibly hazardous, oil occur but ignorance can result in a friendly oil being labelled as harmful. Latin names may sound intimidating but they are the best way to ensure what is in a bottle of essential oil.

Knowing a plant family is also helpful, as plants of the same family have certain common therapeutic properties. For example, the Umbelliferae family includes thyme, fennel, carrot and coriander, which all have digestive and carminative properties. Here is a list of ten plant families covering almost sixty plants whose essential oils are used for aromatherapy:

Burseraceae (resin family): Plants from this family exude resins. Grown mostly in the tropics, common examples are frankincense, myrrh, elemi, benzoin and galbanum. These bring heat, contain energy to move fluids, heal wounds and build the immune system, as well as being excellent meditational aids.

Compositae/Asteraceae (sunflower family): Most of the plants from the Compositae family are known to be healers, anti-inflammatory and sedating to nerves and emotions. Common examples are chamomile, helichrysum (immortelle), tagetes and davana.

Coniferae/Pinaceae (conifer family): Plants from this family include pine, juniper, cypress and cedar, giving oil from wood, needles or cones/berries, etc. They are all strong antiseptics, astringent and diuretic. May irritate skin if used neat.

Graminae/Poaceae (grass family): Grasses give oils that are antiseptic, bactericidal and immune-building, and may be uplifting or grounding. Common examples are lemongrass, citronella, palmarosa and vetiver.

Labiatae/Lamiaceae (mint family): All the oils from the plants of the mint family are therapeutic by nature. Highly odorous, they ease breathing, besides being carminative, immune-builders and mood elevators. Common examples are basil, peppermint, spearmint, sage, rosemary and lavandin.

Lauraceae (laurel family): Common examples are cassia, bay, rosewood, camphor and cinnamon, giving oils from wood, bark or leaves, which are heating, stimulating and enhance memory.

Myrtaceae (myrtle family): Commonly known plants are eucalyptus, tea-tree, clove, cajeput, myrtle, niaouli and nutmeg. All known for their excellent therapeutic effects, they are good antiseptics, decongestants and immune-builders.

Rutaceae (citrus family): This family is known for its fruits and flowers and includes lemon, lime, grapefruit, orange, bergamot orange, mandarin and tangerine. Oils from these plants are highly uplifting, enriching and invigorating.

Umbelliferae/Apiaceae (carrot family): Another therapeutically important plant family including carrots, coriander, fennel, anise, thyme, cumin, caraway, parsley and angelica. Renowned for their digestive and carminative effects, they are good stimulants, digestive tonics, detoxifiers and decongestants.

Zingiberaceae (ginger family): Turmeric, cardamom and ginger are well known representatives of this family. These are spice, root or fruit oils, which increase circulation and heat, and are known as good antiseptics and digestive stimulants.

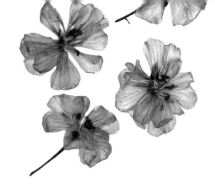

THE TWENTY-FIVE PRINCIPAL ESSENTIAL OILS

Following are the principal essential oils used in aromatherapy for skin, hair and healthcare, along with their detailed profiles.

Note: The predicted benefits of the essential oils mentioned in this chapter are based on the observations of practitioners over many years of practice. Although some essential oils have undergone laboratory testing, many more are yet to be examined scientifically.

Most of the plant oils are known for one or two key properties that can be used on all the systems and organs of the body. If that can be remembered, their use in practice becomes easy. To remember them easily, mark those properties and list them against each plant's name once you have gone through them.

A word to beginners: please go through the cautions indicated for each oil, if any, then mark on a label and stick it to the essential oil bottle, so that every time you use the bottle of essential oil, you are reminded of the precautions you need to take while using that oil.

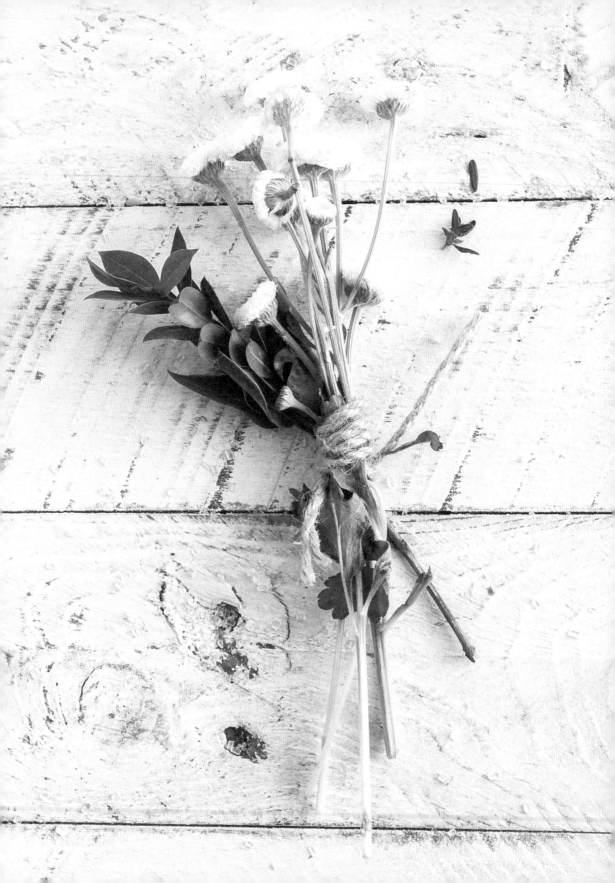

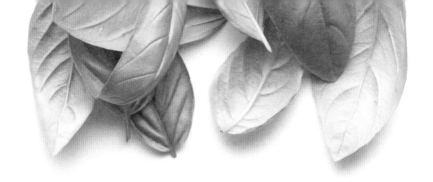

BASIL
(Ocimum basilicum; O. sanctum)

Family: Labiatae/Lamiaceae

There are several varieties of basil. Holy basil (*O. sanctum*) originates in India and is highly revered in spiritual practice. It is considered to be Sattvic (energy of purity) and is widely used in Ayurvedic medicine and healing work. It is known to cleanse the aura, open the heart chakra, promote detachment and bring clarity of mind. Other varieties, such as European or sweet basil (*O. basilicum*), are used more as culinary herbs and contain a higher percentage of methyl chavicol.

Part of the plant used: Leaves, flowering tops

Method of extraction: Steam distillation

Volatility: Top note

Principal constituents: Camphor, cineole, phenol methyl ether, estragole (methyl chavicol), eugenol, linalool and pinene

PROPERTIES, EFFECTS AND METHODS OF USE

Essential oil of basil is a pale yellow liquid with a fresh, sweet-spicy scent, with balsamic undertone. Its odour effect is at first stimulating at first, giving way to a warm, comforting feeling. Basil is an effective diaphoretic (induces perspiration) and also febrifuge (reduces fever) in most colds, flu and lung problems. It is mostly used as a culinary herb; may be taken as a beverage with honey for promoting clarity of mind.

Emotional: Basil is a good fortifier of the nervous system, helps in mental tiredness, fatigue, anxiety and depression. It is particularly useful as a remedy for migraine.

Skin: Fresh leaf juice is used externally for fungal infections on the skin.

Digestive: Basil acts as a tonic and antispasmodic, and is considered to be a good carminative, galactogenic and stomachic. It is also effective for travel sickness and nausea.

Circulatory: Basil stimulates circulation and also clears skin congestion.

Respiratory: Basil is an effective remedy for asthma, bronchitis, nasal polyps and sinusitis.

Muscular: Basil oil is also useful for muscular aches and pains.

Gynaecological: Basil is emmenagogic (regulates the menstrual cycle). It can also be massaged, in a combination, on the solar plexus to control anxiety and menopausal symptoms.

Caution: Avoid during pregnancy; not to be used on sensitive skin; use in the lowest concentrations.

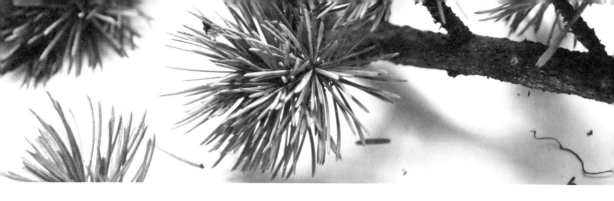

CEDARWOOD
(*Cedrus atlantica; C. deodara*)

Family: Pinaceae

Cedrus, or true cedar, is the genus of four species of evergreen, coniferous, hardy and long-lived trees: *C. atlantica*, the Atlantic or Atlas cedar, is native to the Atlas Mountains of Morocco; *C. libani*, of Lebanon, is native to Syria and south-east Turkey; *C. libani* var. *brevifolia* comes from Cyprus; and *C. deodara*, the deodar, from the Himalayas. Cedars are the trees most mentioned in the Bible, symbolising fertility and abundance. The wood and its oil were used in embalming by the ancient Egyptians. For therapeutic use the only recognised oils of cedar are those from *C. atlantica* or *C. deodara*.

Part of the plant used: Wood

Method of extraction: Steam distillation

Volatility: Middle note

Principal constituents: Terpenic hydrocarbons, a little cedrol (which crystallises when isolated), and sesquiterpenes (50%) – especially cadinene and cedrene

PROPERTIES, EFFECTS AND METHODS OF USE

Cedarwood has an effective therapeutic action on the scalp. In France it is included in commercial shampoos and hair lotions for alopecia. Over the last 100 years, cedarwood's beneficial effects on the skin have been noted and it's highly valued in dermatology. As the oil is considered a sexual stimulant, it could also be used in men's body preparations.

Skin: Cedarwood oil is quite effective for skin problems such as eczema, dermatitis, seborrhoea, rashes, skin eruptions and cellulite.

Hair: Cedarwood oil is also well-known for its therapeutic action for hair and scalp problems including alopecia, falling hair and dandruff. The oil has a tendency to darken hair colour.

Caution: Must not be taken internally. Cedarwood has been prescribed internally in the past as a remedy for haemorrhoids, but stomach problems with intense burning sensations, thirst and nausea were recorded.

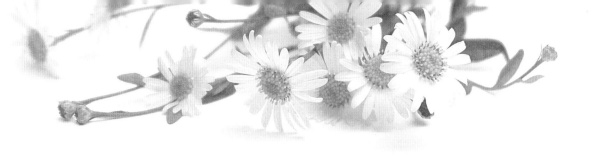

CHAMOMILE, GERMAN
(Matricaria chamomilla)

Family: Compositae/Asteraceae

German chamomile, also known as blue chamomile, yields an oil with a high azulene content, which is used mainly to treat severe skin conditions. This also gives the plant oil a typical blue colour.

Part of plant used: Flowers

Method of extraction: Steam distillation

Volatility: Middle note

Principal constituents: Sesquiterpenes, chamazulene (less than 5%), dihydro-chamazulenes I and II, bisabolenes, sesquiterpenols, sesquiterpenic oxides, lactones and ethers

PROPERTIES, EFFECTS AND METHODS OF USE

Essential oil of German chamomile contains the powerful anti-inflammatory substance azulene, which can relieve a wide variety of skin complaints.

Skin: Anti-inflammatory, soothing and antiseptic; good for sensitive and dry skins; helps to clear acne, eczema, psoriasis, diaper/nappy rash, burns and minor wounds; reduces inflammation. Used in masks, compresses, application or massage.

Digestive: Antispasmodic and anti-inflammatory; soothes diarrhoea, dyspepsia, indigestion, flatulence and colic; restores appetite. Used in compresses, baths, application or massage.

Muscular: Calming and mild analgesic; soothes muscular aches and cramps due to physical exertion; relieves inflammation and pain in rheumatism and arthritis. Used in compresses, baths, application or massage.

Gynaecological: Soothing and antispasmodic; helps painful, heavy or irregular menstruation; relieves premenstrual syndrome and menopausal symptoms. It is also useful for cystitis. Used in compresses, baths or application.

Caution: May cause hypersensitivity if undiluted. Avoid in the first trimester of pregnancy. It may cause skin irritation in some people.

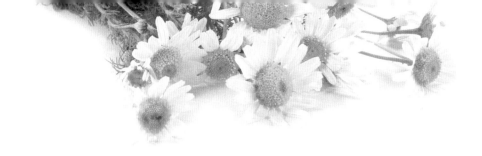

CHAMOMILE, ROMAN
(Chamaemelum nobile)

Family: Compositae/Asteraceae

The small double flower heads of the cultivated variety of this species are dried and then distilled to produce the high-quality oil that is so valuable in aromatherapy practice.

Part of plant used: Flowers

Method of extraction: Steam distillation

Volatility: Middle note

Principal constituent: Esters (75–80%), monoterpinic alcohols (5–6%), ketone-pinocarvone

PROPERTIES, EFFECTS AND METHODS OF USE

Roman chamomile essential oil is highly valued in aromatherapy, its multiple healing properties and low toxicity making it particularly suitable for use on children. Roman chamomile has a light but sharp apple-like aroma and a calming effect on the central nervous system.

Emotional: Calming and relaxing; relieves anxiety, stress, depression, hysteria, irritability and neuralgia; helpful in overcoming neurogenic shock, headaches and insomnia; soothing for children's tantrums. Used in inhalation, vaporisation, baths, application or massage. Useful pre-anaesthetic, preventing postoperative shock.

Skin: Soothing and antiseptic, good for sensitive and dry skins; helps to clear acne, eczema, nappy rash, burns, allergies and minor wounds; reduces inflammation. Used in masks, compresses, application or massage.

Digestive: Antispasmodic; antiparasitic; soothes diarrhoea, dyspepsia, nausea, indigestion, flatulence and colic; restores appetite. Used in compresses, baths, application or massage.

Muscular: Calming and mildly analgesic; soothes muscular aches and cramps caused by physical exertion; relieves inflammation and pain in rheumatism and arthritis. Used in compresses, baths, application or massage.

Gynaecological: Soothing and antispasmodic; helps painful, heavy or irregular menstruation; relieves premenstrual syndrome and menopausal symptoms. Used in compresses, baths or application.

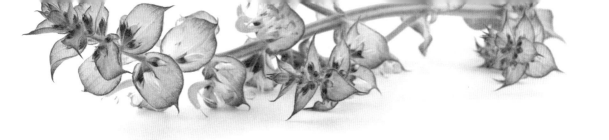

CLARY SAGE
(Salvia sclarea)

Family: Labiatae/Lamiaceae

This beautiful plant is to be found growing high up in the alps wherever the soil is loose and dry. Small blue or white flowers grow out of large, pinky mauve bracts. Branches of these bracts radiate out in pairs from a spectacular central stem that reaches a height of 1.5 metres (60 inches). The powerful aroma of clary sage somewhat resembles that of Muscatel wine; in the past, German winemakers used the herb to improve cheap wines. Clary sage bears no resemblance to common or garden sage, *Salvia officinalis*, which yields an entirely different essential oil.

Part of plant used: Flowering tops

Method of extraction: Steam distillation

Volatility: Top note

Principal constituents: Linalool, linalyl acetate, sclareol, germacrene D, diterpenes, alpha-terpineol

PROPERTIES, EFFECTS AND METHODS OF USE

Clary sage is a neurotonic, powerful relaxant and a sedative. It has a pervading, sweet, sensuous aroma that can be quite heady. The presence of sclareol, which resembles human steroid, is why the oil is known as 'women's best friend' as it is good for all hormonal imbalances, premenstrual syndrome (PMS) and menopausal symptoms.

Emotional: Uplifting and relaxing; helpful in relieving depression, anxiety, tension, mental fatigue and general debility; it is an effective sedative, promoting profound, dream-filled sleep; good for calming cross or irritable children. Used in inhalation, vaporisation, bath, application or massage.

Respiratory: Calming and anti-inflammatory; relieves sore throats and hoarseness. Used in inhalation, vaporisation or application.

Circulatory: An effective remedy for hypertension, the oil is sedative, calming and reduces high blood pressure. Used in inhalation, vaporisation, compresses, baths or massage.

Gynaecological: Antispasmodic, anti-inflammatory and a gentle menstrual stimulant; relieves amenorrhoea, dysmenorrhea, PMS and menstrual pain; helps to establish menstrual regularity; soothes swollen breasts; relieves/prevents hot flushes. Used in compresses, baths or massage.

Caution: Since inhalation of the oil may cause sleepiness, keep to recommended dosages and use for short periods only, preferably at the end of the day when no further physical or mental exertion is required. Do not combine with alcohol or inhale before driving. Avoid use during the first five months of pregnancy.

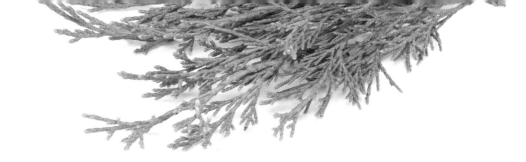

CYPRESS
(Cupressus sempervirens)

Family: Cupressaceae

The elegant, graceful form of this tree is a feature of the landscape of southern France where, traditionally, it is planted in graveyards. Today, C. *sempervirens* is commercially cultivated for its oil in both Germany and France. In the past, the Egyptians used cypress wood to make the coffins in which they placed mummies, while the ancient Chinese believed in the healing properties of the tree, chewing on the fruit to prevent bleeding gums and loss of teeth.

Part of plant used: Twigs, needles, and cones

Method of extraction: Steam distillation

Volatility: Middle note

Principal constituents: Monoterpenes pinene and carene, sesquiterpenes and carvone, 4-terpinol, p-cymene, carveol, cedrol, a-thugene and santene

PROPERTIES, EFFECTS AND METHODS OF USE

Essential oil of cypress is primarily beneficial to the circulatory and vascular systems. It also has both astringent and styptic properties (the latter causes the constriction of blood vessels and helps to staunch bloodloss).

Emotional: Sedative and soothing; helps to clear the mind of grief and prepare it for sleep; useful against insomnia. It can be used in vaporisation, baths, application or massage.

Respiratory: Antispasmodic and antiseptic; relieves spasmodic and whooping coughs, useful for asthma and laryngitis. Used in gargles, inhalation, vaporisation, baths or application.

Skin: Useful for oily skin as an astringent, effective for open pores, it can be used in flower waters, cleansers or facial massage.

Circulatory: Astringent and styptic; relieves fluid retention and cellulite; invaluable in the treatment of bleeding gums, oedema of lower limbs, varicose veins, haemorrhoids, circulatory cramps, chilblains and broken capillaries. Can be used in bath or skin application.

Digestive: Helps in diarrhoea, nausea and dyspepsia.

Muscular: Tonic; helpful for cramps; reduces swelling in rheumatism. Used in baths, compresses, application, or massage.

Gynaecological: Antispasmodic and styptic; can help to staunch a hemorrhage or excessive bloodloss; relieves painful menstruation and menopausal spotting; useful after childbirth as a means of controlling the amount of blood lost and for calming vulval tissues. Used in compresses, baths, application or massage.

Caution: Dilute before use; for external use only. Avoid using if you suffer from high blood pressure.

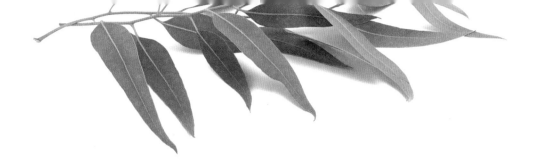

EUCALYPTUS
(Eucalyptus globulus)

Family: Myrtaceae

Of the various species of eucalyptus native to Australia, only a small number are grown for their essential oil. During the heat of summer, eucalyptus trees appear surrounded by a blue haze as essential oil evaporates from their leaves, releasing antiseptic properties that may help to protect against blight and pests. Today, eucalyptus trees are grown successfully in many sub-tropical countries include Spain, Portugal, India, Zimbabwe and China.

Part of plant used: Leaves

Method of extraction: Steam distillation

Volatility: Top note

Principal constituents: An oxide – 1-8-cineole or eucalyptol (60–80%), along with various aldehydes, ketones, sesquiterpinic alcohols and terpenes

PROPERTIES, EFFECTS AND METHODS OF USE

Essential oil of eucalyptus is a strong natural antiseptic that may be effective against a wide range of bacterial and viral infections. It has an overall cooling effect on the body and is useful in reducing fevers. The oil is clear with a strong camphoraceous smell that makes it a good anti-catarrhal and decongestant as well as a good insect repellent.

Emotional: Uplifting and invigorating; clears and stimulates the mind and helps to prevent drowsiness. Used in inhalation, vaporisation, baths application or massage.

Respiratory: Antiseptic and decongestant: helps to fight and prevent colds, flu, throat infections, sinusitis, and headaches caused by congestion; eases tight, dry coughs; relieves the breathlessness of asthma and bronchitis by loosening mucus. Used in gargles, inhalation, vaporisation, baths, application or massage.

Skin: Cooling and antiseptic; effective in the treatment of bacterial/fungal dermatitis, boils, pimples, headlice, and herpes simplex. Used in compresses or application.

Circulatory: Cleansing and detoxifying, it stimulates and strengthens the kidneys. Used in baths, massage or application.

Muscular: Anti-inflammatory, reduces swelling and helps to relieve muscular aches and pains, rheumatism, and arthritis. Can be used in compresses, bath, application or massage.

Urinary: Eucalyptus oil can help to alleviate cystitis when used in a sitz bath.

Caution: Once absorbed into the bloodstream, eucalyptus oil can irritate the kidneys or skin if used in too high a concentration. Do not use on children.

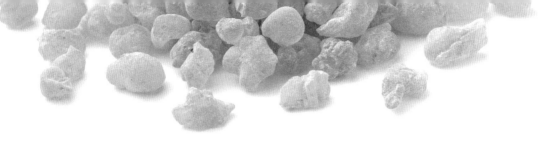

FRANKINCENSE
(Boswellia carterii; B. serrata)

Family: Burseraceae

One of the three gifts from the Magi to the baby Jesus, frankincense has been used since olden times for religious or spiritual rituals and cleansing. Also known as olibanum, this aromatic gum-resin is obtained from trees of the genus *Boswellia*, mainly from *B. carterii*, in Africa and the Middle East and *B. serrata* from various regions of India.

Part of plant used: Exuded gum

Extraction: Steam distillation or solvent extraction

Volatility: Middle note

Principal constituents: Monoterpenes (alpha- and beta-pinene, limonene), sesquiterpine (phellandrene, myrcene), terpinic alcohols, farnesol, borneol, ketonic alcohol (olibbanol)

PROPERTIES, EFFECTS AND METHODS OF USE

A colourless to pale yellow liquid with a warm, balsamic fragrance, subtly lemony, and sometimes with a note of camphor. The odour improves greatly as the oil ages. The odour effect is warming and balancing to the emotions. The oil is considered to be stimulant.

Emotional/mental: Frankincense is a meditational aid, helping to maintain a clear mind and preserve spiritual energy. It relieves nervous depression, stress and anxiety.

Skin: Due to its rejuvenating properties, frankincense is useful in skincare, particularly mature skin, scars and wounds in a massage blend.

Respiratory: Useful for respiratory ailments such as asthma, bronchitis, colds and flu, it can be made into a chest rub.

Gynaecological: Frankincense is a mild hormone regulator, helps in dysmenorrhea and menorrhagia and is useful in the treatment of leucorrhoea and cystitis. Used in compresses, sitz bath, application or massage.

Digestive: It has been found to be useful in dyspepsia and flatulence when diluted in a carrier and rubbed on the abdomen.

Caution: May cause skin irritation in some people.

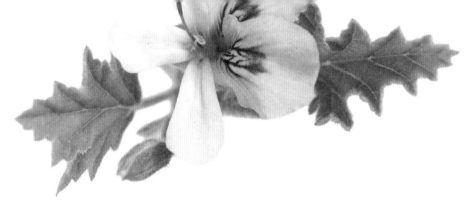

GERANIUM
(Pelargonium graveolens)

Family: Geraniaceae

A native of Africa, the geranium plant was brought to Europe in the late seventeenth century. There are now more than 700 species, of which *P. graveolens* and *P. odoratissimum* are the ones commonly used in aromatherapy. The centre for the commercial cultivation of geranium is the island of Reunion in the Indian Ocean, although France, Spain, Italy, Morocco, Egypt and China are also producers. However, some of the best quality comes from Ooty in South India, and Egypt.

Part of plant used: Leaves

Method of extraction: Steam distillation

Volatility: Middle note

Principal constituents: Mono- and sesqui-terpinol, geraniol, citronellol, linalool and terpinic esters with traces of oxides, ketones and terpenes

PROPERTIES, EFFECTS AND METHODS OF USE

Essential oil of geranium is a good all-rounder. It is anti-infectious, antibacterial, antifungal, antispasmodic and a lymphatic tonic. It is effective in cleansing the body and uplifting the mind. The oil has a rich, sweet aroma and is usually greenish-yellow in colour.

Emotional: Highly versatile. Uplifting as well as relaxing depending on the combination of other oils it is used with. Useful against stress, alleviates depression and anxiety. Used in inhalation, vaporisation, baths, application or massage.

Respiratory: Cleansing and calming; helps to fight colds and flu; relieves throat and mouth infections. Used in mouthwashes or gargles.

Skin: Astringent and balancing; cleanses and tones the skin and normalises secretion of sebum; reduces inflammation; relieves acne, fungal dermatitis, dry eczema, headlice, dandruff, herpes simplex, stretch marks and minor wounds. Soothes measles rashes in children. Used in baths or application.

Digestive: Tonic and cleansing; effective against mouth ulcers, diarrhoea, and gastroenteritis. Used in compresses, baths, application or massage.

Circulatory: Astringent, stimulant and antiseptic; assists elimination of waste products, can help to relieve fluid retention and cellulite. Use in compresses, baths, application or massage.

Gynaecological: Stimulant and regulator of hormone production, it is helpful for premenstrual syndrome, menopausal symptoms, vaginal infections and sterility. Used in compresses, baths, application or massage.

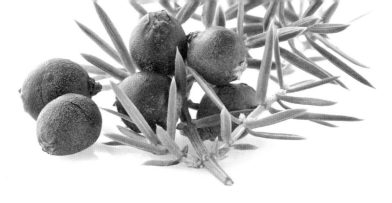

JUNIPER BERRY
(Juniperus communis)

Family: Cupressaceae

Two types of essential oil are distilled from this evergreen shrub. Juniper berry oil is the better quality of the two and the one recommended for aromatherapy use. It is distilled from little ripe berries that have been picked straight from the bush and dried. They are also used during distillation of gin. Occasionally a poorer quality juniper oil is produced by adding berries that have been partially distilled in the making of gin or by extracting oil from the berries, leaves and branches. Both types are sold under the name of juniper berry oil.

Part of plant used: Ripe berries

Method of extraction: Steam distillation

Volatility: Middle note

Principal constituents: Alpha- and beta-pinene, mono- and sesqui- terpineol, and terpenic esters

PROPERTIES, EFFECTS AND METHODS OF USE

Essential oil of juniper berry is noted primarily for its antiseptic and diuretic properties. The oil is colourless to pale yellow when freshly distilled, but it grows darker and thicker with age. The fresh aroma is similar to that of cypress (both plants are from the same family), but sharper and more peppery.

Emotional: Calming and tonic, hypotensive, helpful in overcoming anxiety and mental fatigue. Used in inhalation, vaporisation or application.

Skin: Astringent and cleansing: beneficial for acne, oily skin, greasy hair, dandruff and weeping eczema. Used in masks, compresses or application.

Digestive: Antiseptic and gas/wind relieving: relieves indigestion, flatulence, diarrhoea and colic. Used in baths, compresses, application or massage.

Circulatory: Stimulant and excellent diuretic; helps to lower blood pressure; cleanses the body, relieving fluid retention, cellulite, varicose veins and haemorrhoids; strengthens the kidneys. Used in baths, application or massage.

Muscular: Tonic and stimulant, useful for muscular aches and pains, and rheumatism. Used in compresses, baths, application or massage.

Gynaecological: As a diuretic it's also helpful for irregular or painful menstruation; invaluable when breasts are swollen during menstruation. Use in baths or application. Juniper berry oil may also alleviate cystitis when used in baths or application.

Caution: Avoid use during first five months of pregnancy, and in cases of severe kidney disease. Once absorbed into the bloodstream, the oil can overstimulate the kidneys.

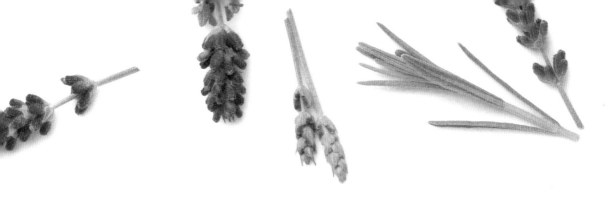

LAVENDER
(Lavandula officinalis;
L. angustifolia)

Family: Labiatae/Lamiaceae

Much of our pure lavender oil now comes from Yugoslavia and Bulgaria; France still produces the finest quality, but production there tumbled with the advent of the hybrid lavandin which grows at low altitudes. True lavender thrives at around 3000 feet (1000 metres). It is the showy purple of lavandin that transforms the landscape of southern France in summer, however the subtle blue of true lavender is far less striking.

Part of plant used: Flowering tops

Method of extraction: Steam distillation

Volatility: Middle note

Principal constituents: Esters 40–55% (including linalyl acetate 30–60%, lavandulyl acetate <6%, geranyl acetate) monoterpenols 27–52% (including linalool and its acetic esters 26–50%, geraniol, terpineol, borneol, lavandulol)

PROPERTIES, EFFECTS AND METHOD OF USE

Lavender essential oil has a balancing and normalising effect, bringing health and harmony to the body and mind. It is non-toxic and has a full, flowery aroma.

Emotional: Uplifting and soothing; alleviates stress, anxiety, depression and general debility; helpful for insomnia, headaches and migraine. Used in inhalation, vaporisation, compresses, baths, application or massage.

Respiratory: Antiseptic and anti-inflammatory, relieves colds, flu, sinusitis and throat infections. Used in inhalation, vaporisation, baths or application.

Skin: Balancing, antiseptic, anti-inflammatory and regenerative; soothes acne, eczema, dandruff, hairloss, headlice, nappy rash, sunburn, insect bites, and boils; relieves athlete's foot and herpes simplex; effective for burns and stretchmarks since it promotes cell growth and helps to minimise scarring. Use in masks, compresses, baths or application. Can also be used neat on insect bites and boils.

Digestive: Cleansing and calming; helps bad breath, mouth ulcers, indigestion, flatulence, nausea and gastroenteritis. Used in compresses, application or massage.

Circulatory: Sedative and decongestant; lowers blood pressure; reduces palpitations; alleviates fluid retention by assisting elimination of waste products through the lymphatic system. Used in baths, application or massage.

Muscular: Analgesic and anti-inflammatory; helpful for muscular sprains, aches, pains and rheumatism. Used in compresses, baths, application or massage.

Gynaecological: Calming and balancing; helps to establish menstrual regularity, good for premenstrual and menopausal symptoms and alleviates thrush. Used in compresses, inhalation, vaporisation, baths, or application.

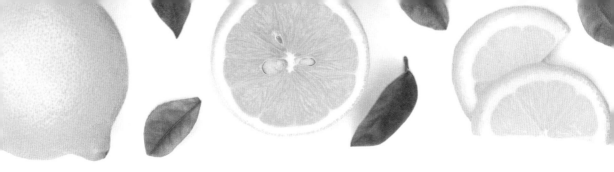

LEMON
(Citrus limonum)

Family: Rutaceae

This member of the citrus family originated in south-east Asia in India, China and Japan, but is now grown extensively in hot countries around the Mediterranean: in Spain, Southern Italy, Sicily and the South of France. Although small, an individual tree can produce up to 1500 lemons per year. Lemon essential oil is called 'polyvalent' (cure-all) by French phytotherapists.

Part of the plant used: Oily rind of the fruit

Method of extraction: Cold expression

Volatility: Top note

Principal constituents: Limonene (up to 90%) camphene, b-pinene, sabinene, myrcene, a-terpinene, linalool, B-bisabolene, nerol and citral (3–5%)

PROPERTIES, EFFECTS AND METHODS OF USE

The therapeutic values of lemon were slow to be recognised. Nicholas Lewery, in his book on simple drugs in 1968, mentioned them. Lemons were classified as digestive, as a blood-cleanser and as helping to sweeten the breath after a heavy meal. They reached the height of their therapeutic fame when they were issued in the British navy to counteract the effects of scurvy due to their vitamin C content (resulting in the erroneous nickname of 'Limey' for the British).

Emotional: Stimulating, uplifting and invigorating; lemon acts to sharpen mind and restore or increase vitality. Used in inhalation, baths (morning) or application.

Digestive: It is a tonic, stimulant, stomachic, carminative, and helps relieve dyspepsia and gastritis.

Respiratory: Lemon is a well-known and popular remedy for colds, bronchitis and laryngitis. Can be used in gargles or application.

Skin: Cooling and cleansing, lemon acts as simple pore-refining toner and is used on greasy skin and blackheads. It soothes itchy skin so helps in psoriasis; makes a good hair rinse for an oily scalp; clears dandruff. Can also be used in application or in a face mask.

Circulatory: Lemon improves circulation so is useful for all vein problems, varicose or broken capillaries. Used in massage or application.

Gynaecological: Lemon also helps the symptoms of premenstrual tensions and insomnia. This is also good for stomach skin during pregnancy, for the breasts and the nipples, improving circulation all around. Used in massage or application.

Caution: Lemon oil should be used fresh as it oxidises quickly if left open or in the light. Oxidised oil can cause a terrible allergic reaction (old oxidised oil will look cloudy – so discard if cloudy). Since lemon is photosensitive it should not be used before going out in the sun or sunbathing.

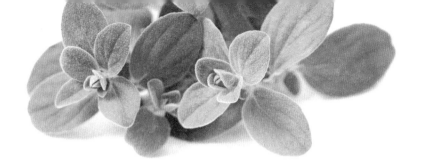

MARJORAM, SWEET
(Origanum majorana)

Family: Labiatae/Lamiaceae

Marjoram is thought to have originated in Asia, but it is being grown all over Europe. The plant was sacred to Indian deities Shiva and Vishnu, and to Osiris in Egypt. To Greeks it was amarakos, a symbol of love and honour. Aphrodite used it to cure the wound of her son, Aeneas; apparently marjoram was scentless until she touched it.

Part of the plant used: Leaves and flowering tops

Method of extraction: Steam distillation

Volatility: Middle note

Principal constituents: Phenols 80% (carvacrol and thymol) with borneol, camphor, cineole, cymene, pinene, sabinene and terpineol

PROPERTIES, EFFECTS AND METHODS OF USE

A pale yellow liquid with a warm, spicy, camphoraceous aroma. Its odour effect is warming and calming; it is reputed to quell sexual desire. Marjoram has always been used as an oil as well as a herb. It's a stomachic, expectorant and sedative, particularly useful when you are tired or suffering from sleeplessness.

Emotional: Marjoram calms and sedates the nerves; it is good for treating insomnia, migraines, nervous tension and tension headaches.

Skin: Useful in ointments for bruises, also in hair formulations to maintain natural colour and lustre of hair and brows.

Digestive: Marjoram is effective in stomach disorders, flatulence and stomach pain. Used in massage or application.

Respiratory: Eases asthma, bronchitis, colds, coughs and snoring. Used in inhalation or vaporisation.

Muscular: Relieves chill pains, muscular stiffness and spasmic pains. Used in massage or application.

Gynaecological: Useful in relieving conditions of painful menstruation, absence of menstruation outside pregnancy and premenstrual syndrome. Quells sexual desire. Used in massage or application.

Caution: Not to be used during pregnancy. It may cause skin irritation in sensitive people.

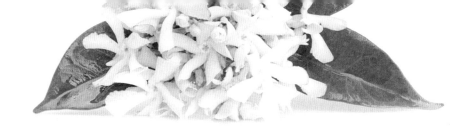

NEROLI
(Citrus aurantium var. *amara)*

Family: Rutaceae

Neroli essential oil is extracted by distillation of the flowers of the bitter orange, also known as the Seville orange. Solvent-extracted absolutes are also available. The main commercial producers are Italy, France, Egypt and Sicily, however the best oil comes from Tunisia and Sicily. Orange flower water is the by-product of the distillation process.

Part of the plant used: Flowers

Method of extraction: Steam distillation

Volatility: Middle note

Principal constituents: Acetic esters, dipentene, terpineol, farnesol, geraniol, indol, jasmone, I-camphene, alpha- and beta-pinene, nerol, nerolidol

PROPERTIES, EFFECTS AND METHODS OF USE

The essential oil is a pale yellow liquid with a sweet, floral fragrance with bitter and sour undertones. The absolute is a dark amber viscous liquid with a fresh warm, sweet-floral fragrance, very similar to the scent of fresh orange blossom. The aroma effect of both neroli and orange flower absolute is uplifting, calming and antidepressant; a reputed aphrodisiac.

Emotional: Neroli is a good relaxing as well as uplifting oil. It gives confidence and strength of mind, and has a slightly hypnotic effect, which helps with sleeplessness. Can be used for inhalation or in a vaporiser.

Skin: Neroli is good for mature skin; also helpful in inflammation, dermatitis and broken capillaries. Used in massage or application.

Respiratory: Neroli oil helps in bronchitis, respiratory disorders and pulmonary tuberculosis. Can be used for inhalation, chest massage or in a vaporiser.

Digestive: Neroli helps in digestive problems like flatulence and enterocolitis and regulates liver and pancreatic malfunctions. Used in massage or application.

Gynaecological: Neroli has a special affinity with the female immune system; it helps women in any stage of transition, reduces cramps and assists in menopause. Used in massage or application.

Caution: Because of neroli's high price, petitgrain is often added to it, which reduces the therapeutic effect of the oil.

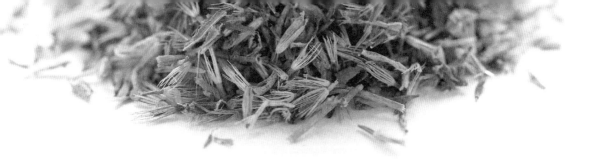

PALMAROSA
(Cymbopogon martinii)

Family: Gramineae/Poaceae

Palmarosa belongs to a family of tropical grasses rich in volatile, aromatic oils, formerly in the genus *Andropogon*, but now included in *Cymbopogon*. Originally from Central and Northern India, and now cultivated in Africa and Madagascar as well, the grass is slender, bearing panicles of blue-white colour that mature to dark red.

Part of the plant used: Leaves and flowers

Method of extraction: Steam distillation

Volatility: Top note

Principal constituent: Monoterpinic alcohols mainly gernaniol (75–90%) and esters

PROPERTIES, EFFECTS AND METHODS OF USE

The plant has long been used in India. Also called poor man's geranium, it is taken internally as a remedy against infection and fever. A high proportion of geraniol in the oil makes it a natural antiseptic and bactericide. Palmarosa can relieve the discomforts of flu and high temperature.

Emotional: Palmarosa has a comparatively mild odour and a relaxing effect on the mind; like geranium it is quite versatile, becoming relaxing in combination with relaxing oils and uplifting in combination with uplifting oils. Used in baths (morning), massage, compresses and application.

Skin: A wonderful remedy for skin conditions like acne because of its natural antiseptic constituents; also works for boils (apply directly), for old acne scars and for wrinkles, especially those occurring after long exposure to the sun. Palmarosa is also useful for hair loss and dandruff control. Baths (morning), massage, compresses and application.

Circulatory: Wonderful remedy for broken veins. Baths (morning), massage, compresses and application.

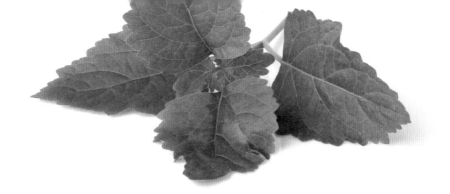

PATCHOULI
(Pogostemon cablin)

Family: Labiatae/Lamiaceae

The essential oil is obtained from the leaves and young shoots of a herbaceous shrub native to Malaysia, where it is called cablin. It is now cultivated extensively, including in India (where it is known as patcha or patchapat), Indonesia, the Seychelles and China. It grows to about three feet in height, and when rubbed the fresh leaves yield the characteristic earthy and woody smell of patchouli. The antiseptic properties of patchouli were studied in 1922 by Gati and Cayol, by Sarbach in 1962 and by many other well-known scientists.

Part of the plant used: Leaves and shoots
Method of extraction: Steam distillation
Volatility: Base note
Principal constituents: Patchoulol and sesquiterpenes

PROPERTIES, EFFECTS AND METHODS OF USE

Patchouli has always played a large part in traditional Malay, Chinese and Japanese medicine, being attributed as a stimulant and bactericidal, effective against fever, epidemics and many other illnesses. It also helps in skin rejuvenation and is used as a remedy for snake venom and insect bites. Patchouli has a great part to play in perfumery as it acts as a natural fixative, reinforcing the woody note in perfume and giving it even greater intensity.

Emotional: Relieves anxieties, tension and restores emotional balance; it is helpful in freeing the mind from past. Being a base note oil, it is used as a natural fixative since its earthy smell lasts longer and becomes quite sensual in combination with the body chemistry; it has also been mentioned in the Kama Sutra. It can be used in inhalation, vaporisation, baths, applications or massage.

Skin: Patchouli is a good tissue regenerator, recommended for many skin conditions: allergies, herpes, impetigo, bedsores, burns, cracked skin, haemorrhoids and eczema. Used in massage or application.

Circulatory: Patchouli is helpful in the treatment of haemorrhoids and varicose veins. Used in massage or application.

Digestive: Patchouli is a good digestive and stomachic; helps in irritable bowel and enterocolitis.

Caution: Patchouli can be adulterated with cubeb and cedar oils. Unless you are sure of the purity of your oil, do not use it therapeutically.

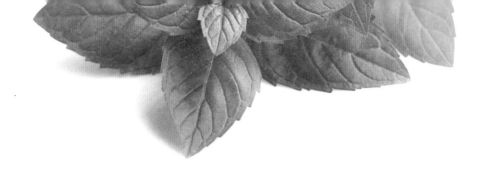

PEPPERMINT
(Mentha x piperita)

Family: Labiatae/Lamiaceae

Commercially cultivated on a wide scale in Europe, USA, and Japan, Peppermint oil is used extensively in the toiletry, food and pharmaceutical industries. A variety of products ranging from toothpastes, mouthwashes and digestive tablets to sweets, ice cream and liquors are flavoured with peppermint. Aromatherapy makes use of a comparatively minute proportion (possibly less than 1%) of the annual worldwide output of peppermint essential oil.

Part of plant used: Leaves

Method of extraction: Steam distillation

Volatility: Top note

Principal constituents: Monoterpinic alcohols: mainly menthol (38–48%); ketones: mainly menthone (20–30%); some monoterpenes and oxides.

PROPERTIES, EFFECTS AND METHODS OF USE

Essential oil of peppermint promotes overall physical and emotional wellbeing, although its healing properties are primarily associated with the digestive system. It is a good antiseptic, antibacterial and antiviral. It has a light, clean, refreshing aroma and is a good insect repellent.

Emotional: Stimulating and strengthening; uplifts the system and is especially useful in the treatment of shock; helpful for neuralgia and relief of general debility, headaches and migraines. Used in inhalation, baths or application.

Respiratory: Probably one of the best remedies for asthma, peppermint is antiseptic and antispasmodic; also effective in reducing mucus and relieving coughs, sinusitis, throat infections, colds, flu and bronchitis. Used in inhalation, baths or application.

Skin: Cooling and cleansing; soothes itchy skin; relieves inflammation. Should be used in dilution for application or massage.

Digestive: Soothing and antispasmodic; relieves acidity, heartburn, diarrhoea, indigestion and flatulence; also highly effective for travel sickness and nausea; helps combat bad breath. Used in gargles or application.

Circulatory: Having a cooling effect, the oil is also helpful for varicose veins and haemorrhoids. Used in compresses or application.

Gynaecological: Cooling and decongestant; encourages menstrual regularity; relieves hot flushes. Used in baths, application or massage. For hot flushes, use orally – just a drop or two in water.

Caution: Too concentrated a dose of peppermint oil can cause itchiness – keep to recommended dilutions. Keep your eyes closed when inhaling. Avoid use if you suffer from epilepsy or other neural disorders.

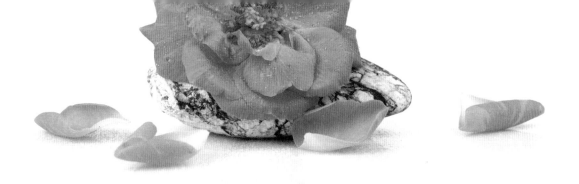

ROSE
(Rosa x *damascena; R.* x *centifolia)*

Family: Rosaceae

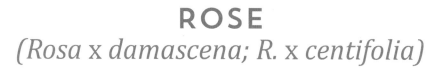

The damask and centifolia roses are hybrids long in cultivation across the world. Rose is highly regarded though it is one of the most difficult oils to extract. It is solvent-extracted, as well as steam-distilled. In the traditional extraction process, almost two tonnes of rose petals are required to obtain a kilogram of rose oil. Because there is hardly any oil in the first distil, distilled water along with oil has to be recycled with fresh petals to increase the oil concentration. The ultimate result is a distiller's dream: rose otto, or *rooh gulab*, as it's called in India (*rooh* meaning lifeforce, *gulab* rose), considered the best quality oil. However, Bulgarian rose oil and absolutes are also popular. Rosewater, the by-product of steam distillation, has been used since the middle ages in skin and beauty care, and also as a flavouring.

Part of the plant used: Flower petals

Method of extraction: Steam distillation

Volatility: Top note

Principal constituents: Eugenol, farnesol and other acids, geraniol (or citronellol), linalool, nerol, nonylic aldehydes, rhodinol and stearoptene

PROPERTIES, EFFECTS, AND METHODS OF USE

Rose is a highly valued essential oil, which alleviates depression and gives a sense of security and spiritual attunement. It keeps your heart open and connected to all things. It reduces anger and strengthens liver function. It is nature's gift to women and alleviates menopausal symptoms. Rose has also been prescribed for frigidity, therefore aphrodisiac properties have been ascribed to it.

Emotional: Rose essential oil is very good for people with a nervous disposition. Its odour effect is calming, uplifting and antidepressant. It is a reputed aphrodisiac. Used in inhalation or application.

Skin: Rose essential oil and rosewater are particularly good for mature skin. Rose oil can be used for skin application or a massage mix. Rosewater or infusions are also useful for eyewashes, eyelid complaints and skin ulcers.

Respiratory: Rose has been found valuable for respiratory problems like coughs, hayfever, sinus congestion and bronchitis. Used in inhalation or application.

Digestive: Rose is a mild laxative and helps in symptoms of anorexia and loss of appetite. In India, rose petals are made into *gulukand*, a paste with honey or sugar, and eaten.

Gynaecological: Rose is considered to be an aphrodisiac and helps in frigidity, premenstrual tension and menopausal symptoms. Used in inhalation or application.

Caution: In spite of its gentle nature, rose oil may sometimes irritate the skin due to its small percentage of eugenol. Also, due to its high price, the purity is always doubtful.

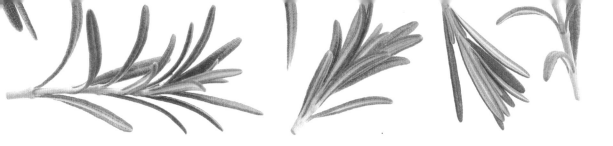

ROSEMARY
(Rosmarinus officinalis)

Family: Labiatae/Lamiaceae

The common name for this plant, rosemary, comes from the Latin *Rosmarinus*, which means 'dew of the sea'. Bushes of this aromatic herb are found growing wild in Mediterranean regions, often quite close to the shore. Its history dates back to the ancient Egyptians, and its revered status as a symbol of love and death to the religious ceremonies and funeral rites of the ancient Greeks and Romans. Therapeutically, it has been in use for hundreds of years, valued for its antiseptic, digestive and invigorating properties.

Part of the plant used: Flowering tops
Method of extraction: Steam distillation
Volatility: Top note
Principal constituents: Pinene, borneol B-pinene, camphor, bornyl acetate, camphene, 1-8 cineole and limonene

PROPERTIES, EFFECTS AND METHODS OF USE

Essential oil of rosemary is noted for its strongly antiseptic and stimulating properties. It is also a gentle analgesic and regulator that helps to balance body and mind. It has a slightly camphoraceous, warm, pungent aroma.
Emotional: Stimulating and astringent; it stimulates the memory, clears the mind, and helps to relieve headaches, migraines, and general fatigue. Used in inhalation, vaporisation, baths, application or massage.

Respiratory: Antiseptic and antispasmodic; relieves coughs, colds and flu. Used in inhalation, compresses or massage.

Skin: Cleansing and stimulating; helps to prevent dandruff and hair loss. Used in rinses, application or massage.

Digestive: Antiseptic and gas/wind relieving; helps indigestion, flatulence, constipation, colitis, gastroenteritis and stomach pains. Also stimulates the liver. Used in compresses, application or massage.

Circulatory: Tonic and astringent; helps in low blood pressure, improves circulation and reduces lymphatic congestion; relieves fluid retention, cellulite and varicose veins. Used in baths, application or massage.

Muscular: Gentle analgesic without sedative effects; relieves general aches and pains, sprains and arthritis. Used in compresses, application or massage.

Gynaecological: Stimulating and normalising; helps to regulate the menstrual cycle. Used in baths, application or massage.

Caution: Avoid use during first five months of pregnancy or if you suffer from high blood pressure.

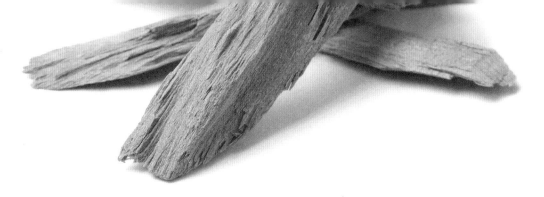

SANDALWOOD
(Santalum album)

Family: Santalaceae

The centre of commercial cultivation of sandalwood is Karnataka in south-west India. From here comes the finest quality essential oil, distilled from the wood of fully mature trees. Sandalwood oil has long been in use in Ayurvedic medicine for its healing properties and is reputed to improve the memory. It is also one of the oils mentioned in the Bible. King Solomon was told by God to use sandalwood for the making of the furniture in his great temple. This he apparently did, and the temple was filled with the beautiful smell of the oil.

Part of plant used: Wood

Method of extraction: Steam distillation

Volatility: Base note

Principal constituents: Santalol (over 90%)

PROPERTIES, EFFECTS AND METHODS OF USE

Sandalwood oil is profoundly relaxing, calming, soothing and a good meditation aid. An excellent antiseptic for both the pulmonary and urinary systems, with a rich woody smell, making the oil quite pleasant for therapeutic use.

Emotional: Calming, sedative and relaxing; beneficial for relieving anxiety and depression; helpful in freeing the mind from the past;

invaluable as a remedy for insomnia. Used in inhalation, vaporisation, baths, application or massage.

Respiratory: Soothing and antiseptic; relieves irritation and soreness in chesty coughs, sore throats and laryngitis; soothes inflammation in bronchitis and asthma. Used in gargles, inhalation, vaporisation, application or massage.

Skin: Balancing and anti-inflammatory; softens dry, mature or wrinkled skin; helps dry dandruff and eczema; reduces inflammation and irritation from sunburn, nettle rash, hives, diaper/nappy rash and allergic conditions. Used in compresses, application or massage.

Digestive: Calming and antispasmodic; subdues vomiting, colic and hiccups; helpful for diarrhoea; soothes heartburn and nausea, especially morning sickness. Used in compresses, application or massage.

Circulatory: Soothing, relieves itchiness in haemorrhoids and varicose veins. Used in compresses or application.

Urinary: Sandalwood oil may soothe cystitis and other urinary infections when used in a sitz bath or application.

Gynaecological: Hormone regulator and balancer, the oil is good for urinary tract infections, premenstrual and menopausal symptoms. Used in baths or application.

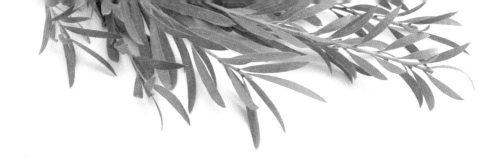

TEA-TREE
(Melaleuca alternifolia)

Family: Myrtaceae

When Captian Cook and his sailors first visited Australia, they were said to have used the leaves of this tree to make a refreshing hot drink. Whether or not they liked the brew is uncertain but the tree has kept the name they gave it. Over the centuries, Aborigines have used tea-tree poultices to cleanse and heal wounds and ulcers. Today it is grown commercially for its oil along the central and northern coasts of New South Wales.

Part of plant used: Leaves

Method of extraction: Steam distillation

Volatility: Top note

Principal constituents: Terpenes, terpinolene, terpinen-4-ol, terpineol

PROPERTIES, EFFECTS AND METHODS OF USE

Tea-tree essential oil is an exceptionally powerful antiseptic, being twelve times as strong as carbolic acid, or phenol, the widely used chemical disinfectant. It has the advantage of being both hypo-allergenic and non-toxic, and may also be effective against a range of bacterial, viral and fungal conditions. The oil can be pale green to almost water-clear, and its aroma is an effective insect repellant.

Respiratory: Bactericidal and antiviral; helps to fight colds and flu; alleviates sore throats, tonsillitis and gum disease; eases bronchitis, chesty coughs and congestion. Used in gargles, mouthwashes, compresses, inhalation, vaporisation or application.

Skin: Cleansing, cooling and antifungal; relieves boils and rashes; soothes sunburn; encourages open, cracked skin and wounds to heal while protecting it from infection; relieves athlete's foot and nail bed infections. Used in masks, compresses, foot or hand baths or application.

Digestive: Bactericidal, antiviral, and antifungal; eases mouth ulcers; calms diarrhoea and relieves gastroenteritis. Used in mouthwashes, compresses, application or massage.

Gynaecological: Very effective for genital infections, especially leucorrhoea and candida (thrush). Used in sitz baths, douches, baths or application.

Caution: Although this oil can be used neat, it may sometimes cause sensitisation of the skin.

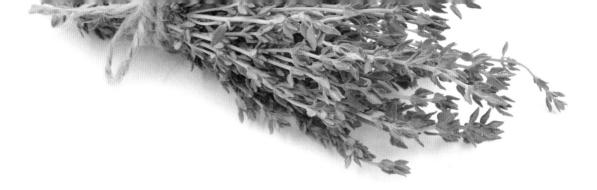

THYME
(Thymus vulgaris; T. citriodorus)

Family: Labiatae/Lamiaceae

The name 'thyme' comes from the Greek word *thymos*, meaning smell, because of the fragrance of the plant. Thyme belongs to a genus of over 300 species of hardy, perennial herbaceous plants and shrubs that are native to Europe, particularly around the Mediterranean. It is one of Hippocrates's 400 simple remedies.

Part of plant used: Leaves and flowering tops

Method of extraction: Steam distillation

Volatility: Top note

Principal constituents: 25–40% thymol and carvacrol with borneol, cineole, linalool, menthone, p-cymene, pinene and triterpenic acid

PROPERTIES, EFFECTS AND METHODS OF USE

Thyme has been used differently by different cultures. The Romans used it medicinally; the ancient Egyptians called it 'tham' and used the plant in embalming. The Greeks knew of two types: Dioscorides, the Greek physician and author of *De Materia Medica*, talked of white, used for medicinal purposes, and black, which was not favoured as it 'corrupted the organism and provoked the secretion of bile'. Thyme is well-known for its digestive properties.

Emotional: During the eighteenth century it was recommended for nervous disorders as it strengthens the nervous system and re-establishes strength in convalescence.

Digestive: The digestive properties of thyme have been known since olden times, and infusions of the herb were consumed at the end of banquets for digestive purposes. It is a tonic, stimulant, stomachic and digestive; it relieves gastritis, enterocolitis and mouth thrush. Can be used in gargles, compresses and application.

Respiratory: It is a useful oil for respiratory infections, asthma and bronchitis. Used in vaporisors, inhalation and application.

Muscular: Thyme is effective for treating swellings provoked by gout or rheumatic problems, for joint pains, backache and sciatica. Used in application or massage.

Gynaecological: Thyme oil is useful for urinary and vaginal infections, endometritis (candida), prostatitis and vaginitis; can be used in a douche or sitz bath.

Caution: May cause skin irritation in sensitive people.

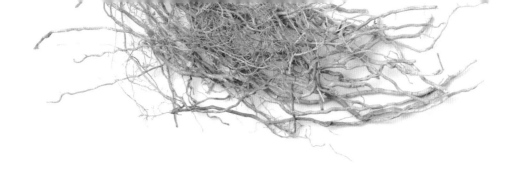

VETIVER; VETIVERT
(Chrysopogon zizanioides)

Family: Gramineae/Poaceae

The essential oil known as vetiver is derived from vetiver grass. It is cultivated in tropical and subtropical climates. The grass, a close relative of other aromatic grasses such as lemongrass, is upright with narrow odourless leaves – it is the roots that have a strong scent, similar to sandalwood or violets. In India, vetiver is known as 'khus'. The grass has to be at least two years old before the roots can be dried in the hot sun.

Part of the plant used: Root

Method of extraction: Steam distillation

Volatility: Base note

Principal constituent: An alcohol called vetiverol and vetiveryl acetate

PROPERTIES, EFFECTS AND METHOD OF USE

Vetiver oil is dark brown with a warm peppery, spicy, woody earthy smell. Renowned as 'the oil of tranquillity', vetiver imparts a sense of calm and peacefulness. It is therefore ideal in times of stress, tension and physical or mental exhaustion. In beauty care, vetiver enables the skin to retain water more readily, making it one of nature's best moisturisers.

Emotional: Calming and relaxing; beneficial for relieving stress, tension, physical or mental exhaustion; especially effective in post-partum depression. Used in inhalation, vaporisation, baths, application or massage.

Skin: Soothing and moisturising, vetiver oil plumps out the tissues of the skin and helps to bring back a more youthful softness to mature skin. Used in a massage blend. When massaged on the breasts, it holds moisture and helps plump out wrinkes.

Digestive: The oil helps clear liver congestion. Used in compress or application.

Gynaecological: The oil is a female tonic and hormone regulator, relieves amenorrhoea. Can be used in sitz bath or application.

Caution: Beware of oils adulterated with synthetics, as the adulterated versions have a noxious effect on the skin.

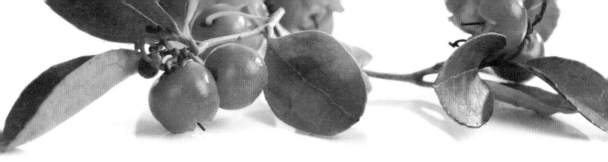

WINTERGREEN
(Gaultheria procumbens)

Family: Ericaceae

This evergreen flowering shrub, native to the United States and Canada, is also found in mountainous areas of the Indian subcontinent. In America, it also called 'partridge berry' or 'checkerberry' and has been used by Native Americans for its remarkable therapeutic properties. They masticated the leaves when they had pain or fever, prepared refreshing drinks with them, and also fed the berries to their animals.

The leaves of the plant have to be macerated for up to 24 hours in hot water to produce the fermentation that releases the essentials of the plant.

Part of the plant used: Leaves

Method of extraction: Maceration/distillation

Volatility: Top note

Principal constituents: 90–95% methyl salicylate, ketone, secondary alcohol and an ester

PROPERTIES, EFFECTS AND METHOD OF USE

Renowned for its anti-rheumatic properties, the oil is colourless but when it ages becomes reddish brown. It has a characteristic camphoraceous smell noticeable in most pain balms and liniments, however, synthetic methyl salicylate is used often as less expensive.

Emotional: Highly aromatic and reminiscent of camphor with a note of vanillin, the aroma provides mental clarity, relieves mental fatigue and is helpful in headaches and migraines. Used in inhalation, vaporisation and application.

Respiratory: The strong aroma helps to clear nasal, sinus and bronchial congestions. Used in inhalation, vaporisation and application.

Muscular: The oil is renowned for its anti-rheumatic properties and its beneficial effect on the muscular system; it helps in gout and stiffness due to old age. Even the leaves of the plant can be warmed up and applied as poultices for muscular and rheumatic swellings. Used in massage or compresses.

Circulatory: Wintergreen has a diuretic effect and helps circulation and decongestion of lymphatics. It can also be used in the treatment of cellulite in combination with other oils. Used in massage or application.

Gynaecological: The oil is a stimulant and emmenagogue, and also relieves menstrual cramps. Used in massage or compresses.

Caution: Methyl salicylate is often sold as wintergreen oil, so check with your source. Methyl salicylate, being a chemical, may cause skin sensitisation if applied directly.

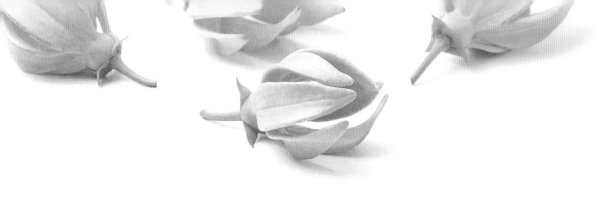

YLANG YLANG
(Cananga odorata var. *genuina)*

Family: Annonaceae

This essential oil is produced by water or steam distillation of the flowers of tall, tropical trees from Asia, commonly called cananga. Most ylang ylang is produced in Madagascar, the Phillipines and the Comoro Islands. There are four grades of ylang ylang: 1, 2, 3 – and a ylang ylang extra, which is more expensive and has a superior fragrance. The islanders used the oil on their body during the rainy season to protect themselves from contagious illnesses and infections. Some used to mix the oil with coconut oil and apply to the hair before entering the sea, to protect it.

Part of the plant used: Fresh flowers

Method of extraction: Steam distillation

Volatility: Middle note

Principal constituents: Alpha pinene, sesquiterpenes – cadinene, caryophyllene, benzoic acid, cresol, eugenol, 5–7% linalyl acetate, 8–10% linalyl benzoate, 30–32% linalool and geraniol

PROPERTIES, EFFECTS AND METHODS OF USE

Ylang ylang is a pale yellow liquid with an intensely sweet, floral scent reminiscent of a blend of jasmine and almonds. The oil has been found to be anti-infectious and has a good result in malaria, typhus and other fevers.

Emotional: Ylang ylang is a sedative, helping to calm the nerves, and a good hypotensive; it reduces palpitations, hypertension and high blood pressure. Its odour effect is intoxicating and antidepressant; a reputed aphrodisiac and a good support for fidgidity. Can be used for inhalation, vaporisation or massage.

Skin and hair: Ylang ylang promotes hair growth and controls dandruff. It can be used in skin formulations to tan the skin (avoid overexposure to the sun). Used in application or massage.

Respiratory: The anti-infectious properties of the oil help in respiratory and pulmonary infections. Used in inhalation or vaporisation.

Circulatory: The oil reduces hypernoea (over-accelerated breathing rate) and tachycardia (abnormal rapidity of heartbeat). It is a good hypotensive and helps reduce blood pressure. Used in inhalation, vaporisation or massage.

Digestive: Ylang ylang is an antispasmodic and antiseptic for intestinal infections, diarrhoea and flatulence. Used in compress or application.

Gynaecological: A balancer of the female immune system, it helps in premenstrual syndrome, reducing negative emotions, tensions, cramps and headaches.

Caution: The oil is extracted in many stages and many fractions are taken out; all qualities are sold as ylang ylang so try to buy only from a trusted source. Do a skin test before use as certain varities can cause skin irritation.

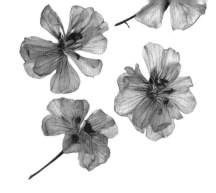

OTHER IMPORTANT ESSENTIAL OILS

AJWAIN *(Trachyspermum ammi)*
Family: Umbelliferae/Apiaceae

Source: Also known as ajowan, bishop's weed and Indian thyme, ajwain is native to India, but also cultivated in Iran, Egypt, Pakistan and Afghanistan. The oil is extracted from the seeds through steam distillation.

Principal constituents: Thymol (22.58%)

Aromatherapy uses: Ajwain oil has insecticidal, antibacterial, antifungal, anti--oxidant, antimicrobial, anti-inflammatory, anti-filarial, nematicidal, anthelmintic, hypotensive, analgesic and antitussive properties. Ajwain seeds contain ethanol and acetone extracts, which have antibacterial anti-filarial properties.

Description and odour effect: Ajwain is a herbaceous annual, 30–70 centimetres in height, bearing feathery leaves and red flowers. The oil is a pale yellowish-brown, and thin. It has a herbaceous, spicy, medicinal odour, with a strong top note similar to thyme.

Caution: Dilute before use; for external use only. May cause skin irritation in some individuals: a skin test is recommended prior to use. Contact with eyes should be avoided.

ANGELICA *(Angelica archangelica)*
Family: Umbelliferae/Apiaceae

Source: The essential oil is obtained by steam distillation of roots or seed from a plant native to Europe and Siberia.

Principal constituents: Angelicin, bergaptene, phellandrenic compounds and other terpenes.

Aromatherapy uses: Psoriasis, arthritis, rheumatism, respiratory ailments, fatigue, nervous tension, cold and flu. Can be used in inhalation, vaporisation, application or massage.

Description and odour effect: The root oil is colourless, turning yellow then dark yellow as it ages. It has a rich earthy herbaceous scent. The seed oil is colourless and has a fresher, spicy top note. The odour effect of both oils is stimulating and aphrodisiac.

Caution: The root oil (not seed oil) should not be applied to the skin shortly before exposure to sunlight as it may cause pigmentation. Avoid during pregnancy.

ANGELICA ROOT *(Angelica sinensis)*
Family: Umbelliferae/Apiaceae

Source: Angelica is a large hairy, biennial plant with ferny leaves and white flowers that can grow 1.5 to 2.5 metres tall. It is commonly known as dong quai or 'female ginseng'; *A. sinensis* grows high in the mountains of China, Japan, and Korea where it was traditionally used. The oil is extracted from the roots by steam distillation and CO_2 extraction.

Principal constituents: Ligustilide and bergaptene.

Aromatherapy uses: In Chinese medicine, angelica is used to soothe menopausal symptoms and negative moods, as well as for its skin-enhancing properties. It relieves cramps and spasms.

Angelica root oil is a good bactericidal. It can also be used to relieve mental exhaustion, as well as dry skin conditions. Its rich herbaceous aroma gives it great strength in diffusion.

Description and odour effect: A clear, red-brown liquid with medium viscosity, which is rich, herbaceous, musky, warm, and slightly spicy with a base note and medium aroma.

Caution: This oil is phototoxic due to the presence of bergaptene, so avoid direct exposure to sunlight for up to 12 hours. Dilute before use; for external use only. May cause skin irritation in some individuals. Contact with eyes should be avoided.

ANISEED/ANISE *(Pimpinella anisum)*
Family: Umbelliferae/Apiaceae

Source: The essential oil is distilled from the seed fruits of a tender annual plant from south-west Asia. Also known as sweet cumin.

Principal constituents: Anethole 80–90% with little aldehyde, anisic acid and methyl chavicol.

Aromatherapy uses: The main property of anise is digestive, in premenstrual tension and menopausal symptoms. The herb is used mostly as a tisane, as it helps with indigestion due to anxiety and nervousness, and relaxation after a meal.

Description and odour effect: The oil is colourless or pale yellow, smells very sweet and very characteristic, a little like fennel.

Caution: The essential oil is strong and toxic – could be dangerous for the nervous system.

BERGAMOT *(Citrus bergamia)*
Family: Rutaceae

Source: Obtained by expression of the rind of the small orange-like fruit native to Italy.

Principal constituents: Up to 50% linalyl acetate, bergamotine, bergaptene, d-limonene and linalool.

Aromatherapy uses: Colds and flu, fever, infectious illness, tonsillitis (a few drops in water to be used as gargle). Also, anxiety and depression. Can be used in inhalation, vaporisation, application or massage.

Description and odour effect: A light green essence with a delightful citrus aroma and a hint of spice. Refreshing and uplifting to the emotions.

Caution: Not to be used on the skin shortly before exposure to sunlight as it may cause pigmentation. Alternatively for skin application try to obtain rectified bergamot oil (called 'Bergamot FCF'), which is free of bergaptene (the substance that causes skin pigmentation). Whole bergamot oil can be used as a room scent.

BENZOIN *(Styrax benzoin)*
Family: Styracaceae

Source: Steam distillation of the gum resin exudes from the bark of the tree native to Laos and Vietnam but now grown in and around Malaysia, Java and Sumatra.

Aromatherapy uses: Skincare (particularly for eczema and psoriasis), frostbite, bedsores, wounds and skin ulcerations; also useful for catarrh and chest infections. Used in application or massage.

Description and odour effect: A colourless to pale yellow liquid with a strong vanilla-like fragrance.

Principal constituents: 20–25% cinnamic acid, vanillin, coniferyl benzoate, benzoic acid, phenyl ethylene and phenyl propyl alcohol.

Caution: Mostly available as solvent-extracted absolute or resinoid – may irritate the skin; do a patch test before using on the skin.

BIRCH *(Betula pendula)*
Family: Betulaceae

Source: The birch is a graceful tree with a pyramidal shape. It has bright green leaves and dark reddish-brown aromatic bark, which is broken into plates. Native to southern Canada and southeastern USA; it now also grows in Russia and parts of Eastern Europe. The oil is extracted from the bark through steam distillation.

Principal constituents: Methyl salicylate (up to 97%).

Aromatherapy uses: Prevents bacterial and fungal infections. Aids diabetes management. Reduces pain in the joints and muscles. It also relieves symptoms of arthritis as it stimulates the circulatory system and improves circulation.

Description and odour effect: Birch has a sweet, sharp, camphoraceous aroma that is fresh and smells like wintergreen. The oil is a thin, colourless to pale-yellow liquid.

Caution: Dilute before use; for external use only. May cause skin irritation in some individuals; a skin test is recommended prior to use. Contact with eyes should be avoided.

BLACK PEPPER *(Piper nigrum)*
Family: Piperaceae

Source: Steam distillation of the dried peppercorns from a woody vine native to south-west India. Most of the oil is produced in India, although it is also distilled in Europe and the USA from imported peppercorns.

Principal constituents: Monoterpenes (limonene, pinene), sesquiterpenes (myrcene, phellandrene, beta-caryophyllene, beta-bisabolene, sabinene, camphene and alpha-terpenene), few alcohols (linalool, pinocarveol, alpha-terpineol), ethers, ketones, aldehydes, acids and selenium.

Aromatherapy uses: Poor circulation, muscular aches and pains, loss of appetite, nausea, colds and flu, infections and viruses, lethargy, mental fatigue. It is diaphoretic, carminative, aperient, antispasmodic, antirheumatic, antiarthritic and antibacterial. Can be used in baths, vaporisation, massage or application.

Description and odour effect: A pale, greenish-yellow liquid with a hot, spicy, piquant odour. The smell is stimulating and warming; a reputed aphrodisiac.

Caution: Use in a low concentration; avoid on sensitive skin as the oil can irritate skin.

CADE *(Juniperus oxycedrus)*
Family: Cupressaceae

Source: Steam distillation of young twigs and wood from the Mediterranean equivalent of the common juniper.

Principal constituents: Phenol (creosol guaiacol), sesquiterpenes (cadinene) and other terpenes.

Aromatherapy uses: Pure oil is one of the best remedies for hair loss, dandruff, hair weakened by dyeing and bleaching, and skin eruptions. Use it for massage or application.

Description and odour effect: The oil is resinous, darkish brown/black in colour, and has a strange waxy smell that is even caustic and tarlike.

Caution: Cade is often adulterated with pine, birch petrol and tar, so be sure of the quality. Adulterated oil can provoke severe skin reactions.

CAJUPUT *(Melaleuca leucadendron)*
Family: Myrtaceae

Source: With a name derived from Malay 'kayu-puti or caju-puti', meaning 'white trees', this species is from the same family as tea-tree and niaouli. The young twigs, leaves and buds are fermented before distillation.

Principal constituents: Cineole (40–70%), alpha-pinene, beta-pinene, limonene, alpha terpinene, alpha terpineol, gamma terpinene, terpinolene and terpineol, along with aldehydes like benzoic, butyric and valeric.

Aromatherapy uses: Useful oil for rheumatism and stiff joints; also a valuable treatment for cystitis. Can also be used for bursitis, chest infections, colds, cough, hayfever, headaches, sore throat etc. Can be used in application, massage, inhalation and gargles.

Description and odour effect: Oil is colourless to pale with a camphoraceous, spicy aroma which helps clear nasal congestion and headaches.

Caution: Should not be used internally.

CALAMUS ROOT *(Acorus calamus)*
Family: Acoraceae

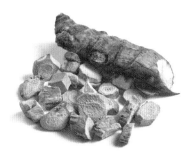

Source: This perennial plant with greenish berries is indigenous to theprotected swampy ditches and marshes of the northern hemisphere. Also known as sweet flag, it was well-known in Biblical times and mentioned as one of the ingredients of the holy anointing oil. In Ayurvedic tradition it is known as vacha. Mostly from India, the oil is extracted from the roots of the plant through steam distillation.

Principal constituents: Asarone up to 78%.

Aromatherapy uses: Anti-rheumatic and anti-arthritic. This oil is particularly stimulating for the nerves and blood circulation. Essential oil of calamus is known for its antispasmodic properties. Antibiotic: due to its toxic nature, calamus essential oil does not allow any biotic growth and acts as a natural antiseptic. Cephalic: this essential oil has a refreshing effect on the brain and enhances memory. It is also used as an aphrodisiac.

Description and odour effect: A slightly viscous, pale yellow to brown liquid with a faintly sweet, waxy scent with a base note and medium aroma.

Caution: For external use only. May cause skin irritation in some individuals: a skin test is recommended prior to use. Contact with eyes should be avoided.

CAMPHOR, BORNEOL *(Dryobalanops aromatica* syn. *D. camphora)*
Family: Dipterocarpaceae

Source: Steam distillation of an evergreen plant native to the west coast of Sumatra and the north of Borneo.

Principal constituents: Terpinic alcohol, borneol and isobornyl acetate

Aromatherapy uses: Borneol camphor has been valued in Ayurvedic medicine for many centuries. It is used in combination with other plants for eye injuries, infections, headaches and migraines. It is considered good for insect and snakebites, inflammations, muscular and rheumatic pain, and cuts and bruises. A diuretic, it is renowned as a tonic for the kidneys. A strong antiseptic, it helps in leucorrhoea and vaginitis. Can be used in application and massage.

Description: Smells primarily of camphor, the oil is pale yellow and does not crystallise easily. It is only the borneol in the oil that crystallises in small grains or thin layers of oil.

Caution: Do not use camphor with homeopathic medicines; it will affect their efficacy.

CAMPHORWOOD *(Cinnamomum camphora)*
Family: Lauraceae

Source: Steam distillation of the clippings, wood and root of an evergreen tree native to China, Taiwan and Japan. The older the tree, more the oil it contains.

Principal constituents: Azulene, borneol, cadinene, camphene, carvacrol, cineole, cuminic alcohol, dipentene, eugenol, phellandrene, pinene, sajrol and terpineol.

Aromatherapy uses: The oil is good for inflammation, muscular and rheumatic pain, and cuts and bruises; also used as an insect repellent. Can be used for application or massage.

Description: Crystalline ketone camphor ($C_{10}H_{16}$) or solid camphor is a pale yellow oil.

CARAWAY *(Carum carvi)*
Family: Umbelliferae/Apiaceae

Source: Steam distillation from a plant native to south eastern Europe.

Principal constituents: 50–60% carvone; others are carvacol, carvene and limonene. Research has confirmed that a high percentage of carvone helps in digestion, stimulation and release of gastric juices.

Aromatherapy uses: Caraway is excellent for all digestive problems such as flatulence, pain, dyspepsia, colic and colitis. The oil is also considered to be a mild antiseptic and an effective remedy for vertigo. Used in application and massage.

Description and odour effect: The oil is sometimes tinged with yellow, which darkens as the oil matures. The smell is muskier than cumin, fruitier and hotter.

Caution: Due to its high ketone content, the oil should be used with caution as it can be neurotoxic for certain people.

CARDAMOM
(Elettaria cardamomum)
Family: Zingiberaceae

Source: Steam distillation of the dried ripe fruit (seeds) from a reed-like herb native to Asia.

Principal constituents: Cineole, alpha terpinyl acetate and terpineol, with a little limonene.

Aromatherapy uses: Digestive disturbances, boosts metabolism, controls nausea and vomiting, mental fatigue, nervous exhaustion. Prevents microbial infections. Can be used in inhalation, vaporisation, application or massage.

Description and odour effect: A colourless to yellowish liquid with a sweet-spicy, warming fragrance. The odour effect is warming and stimulating; a reputed aphrodisiac.

Caution: Use in the lowest concentration as it has a high odour intensity.

CARROT SEED
(Daucus carota)
Family: Umbelliferae/Apiaceae

Source: Carrot is native to Europe and southwestern Asia. It is a biennial plant that grows a rosette of leaves with an umbel of white flowers that produce the seeds. The name is derived from the Greek *carotos*, for healing. The oil is extracted from the seeds by steam distillation.

Principal constituents: Cineol and caratol.

Aromatherapy uses: Carrot seed oil is full of naturally occurring beta-carotene and carotenoids, so ideal for mature or dry skin types, as well as damaged and brittle hair. Also used for digestive purposes.

Description and odour effect: It is a pale yellow to amber liquid with a thin viscosity. Fragrance is a middle note with a medium aroma, this oil has a strong woody, earthy and musky scent.

Caution: For external use only. May cause skin irritation in some individuals; a skin test is recommended prior to use. Contact with eyes should be avoided.

CASSIA
(Cinnamomum cassia)
Family: Lauraceae

Source: Also known as bastard cinnamon and Chinese cinnamon, cassia's first recorded use in China dates back to the Han Dynasty (200 BCE–200 CE). The oil is extracted from the leaves of the plant through steam distillation.

Principal constituents: Cinnamic aldehyde, benzaldehyde, linalool, methyl chavicol and cinnamyl acetate.

Aromatherapy uses: The essential oil of cassia has various benefits to the digestive system and treats diarrhoea. Anti-emetic. This oil can also be used to treat nausea and to stop vomiting. It is an antidepressant, as the essential oil fights depression and uplifts mood.

Description and odour effect: It is a transparent pale yellow to reddish liquid having a pungent, warm aroma. It has a strong top note.

Caution: For external use only. May cause skin irritation; contact with eyes should be avoided.

CATNIP *(Nepeta cataria)*
Family: Labiatae/Lamiaceae

Source: Catnip is also referred to as catmint and has earned the reputation of having an intoxicating effect on house cats, due to a compound that causes temporary euphoria. The catnip plant is widely used in commercial tea and in cat toys and is cultivated in parts of Canada such as Alberta and British Columbia. Oil is extracted from the whole plant through steam distillation.

Principal constituents: Nepetalactone (78–85%).

Aromatherapy uses: Catnip oil is stomachic, meaning that it keeps the stomach in order and functioning well. It cures stomach disorders and ulcers, while ensuring the proper flow of bile and gastric juices and acids in the stomach.

Description and odour effect: A clear yellow to light brown liquid with a thin consistency. The aroma of the oil is basically green and herbaceous with sweet floral hints.

Caution: Do not ingest. For external use only. May cause skin irritation in some individuals; use in dilution only. Contact with eyes should be avoided.

CELERY *(Apium graveolens)*
Family: Umbelliferae/Apiaceae

Source: From a hardy biennial vegetable grown for its crisp, long crescent-shaped stalks, the oil can be extracted from all parts but the oil from its seeds is preferred for therapeutic use.

Principal constituents: Lactone sedanolide, palminic acid and terpinic hydrocarbons – limonene and selinene.

Aromatherapy uses: Hippocrates and Dioscorides thought of it as a strong diuretic. Also used for chilblains. It can be used as a raw or cooked vegetable. Particularly good for diabetics who suffer from hypoglycaemia. It is also considered to be a good aphrodisiac. Celery juice helps in cystitis besides helping in menstrual complaints.

Description and odour effect: Celery seed oil is a pale yellow liquid with a strong celery aroma.

Caution: Celery is allergenic, especially the seeds. It can provoke severe allergic reactions. For people with celery allergy, exposure can be potentially fatal.

CINNAMON BARK
(Cinnamomum verum syn. *C. zeylanicum)*
Family: Lauraceae

Source: Steam distillation of the bark chips from the small tree native to Sri Lanka, India and Madagascar. A low-grade oil is obtained from the leaves and twigs.

Principal constituents: Cinnamic aldehyde (60–70%), caryophyllene, cymene, eugenol, linalool, pinene, etc.

Aromatherapy uses: Cinnamon is highly microbial and can be used in a vaporiser as an antiviral fumigant during infectious illness. It's also useful as antidepressant, room scent or as an antibiotic. Taken as a tisane, cinnamon is good for circulation, detoxifies and helps burn fat, besides helping to regulate blood sugar level.

Description and odour effect: A light amber liquid with a sweet, warm-spicy, dry, tenacious aroma. The odour effect is stimulating and warming; a reputed aphrodisiac.

Caution: This oil is a powerful skin irritant. Use only in a minute quantity in dilution; otherwise use only as a room scent.

CITRONELLA *(Cymbopogon nardus)*
Family: Gramineae/Poaceae

Source: Citronella oil is extracted from a tall grass native to India, Sri Lanka and Java. It is a very aromatic perennial that grows to nearly a metre in height. Oil is extracted by steam distillation of the leaves.

Principal constituents: Citronellal, citral, citronellol, geraniol.

Aromatherapy uses: All-natural insect repellent. Anti-inflammatory and pain reducer. Like many citrus essential oils, it is uplifting and stress reducing. Kills external parasites.

Description and odour effect: A top note aroma, the oil is clear light yellow to brownish liquid. Citronella has a well-rounded citrus note.

Caution: For external use only. May cause skin irritation in some individuals and contact with eyes should be avoided.

CLOVE BUD *(Eugenia caryophyllus)*
Family: Myrtaceae

Source: Water distillation from the buds of the slender evergreen tree native to Indonesia. Most supplies of the oil are from Madagascar. Lower grades of clove oil are distilled from the leaves and stems.

Principal constituents: Phenols (70–80%) particularly eugenol, acetyl eugenol, benzoic acid, benzyl benzoate and furfurol.

Aromatherapy uses: It is employed as a first aid measure for toothache (the oil is analgesic), but should never be used long-term as it is a skin irritant and will damage the gums. While awaiting dental treatment, a single drop of the oil can be dropped into the tooth cavity or rubbed into the gums. Oil can be vaporised as a room scent, or used as a fumigant during infectious illness. Besides direct application for toothache, the oil can be used in vaporisation and blended with other oils for application and massage.

Description and odour effect: A light amber liquid with a bittersweet spicy aroma. The odour effect is warming and stimulating. A reputed aphrodisiac.

Caution: The oil is a powerful skin irritant due to its high eugenol content. Use in dilution or only as a room scent. Use in the lowest concentration as it has a high odour intensity. It should be stored in glass containers as it will corrode an aluminium container.

CORIANDER *(Coriandrum sativum)*
Family: Umbelliferae/Apiaceae

Source: Steam distillation of the herb native to Europe and western Asia. Most of the oil is produced in Eastern Europe.

Principal constituents: An alcohol (coriandrol, 60–65%), geraniol and pinene.

Aromatherapy uses: Arthritis, muscular aches and pains, poor circulation, digestive problems, colds and flu, mental fatigue and nervous exhaustion. Can be used as a compress or in a massage mix.

Description and odour effect: A colourless to pale yellow liquid with a sweet, spicy, faintly musky aroma. It has a stimulating, warming aroma and is a reputed aphrodisiac.

CUBEB *(Piper cubeba)*
Family: Piperaceae

Source: Cubeb essential oil is extracted from the cubeb plant, which mostly grows in Java and Sumatra. Also known as Java pepper, tailed pepper or shi-tal chini/kabab chini in India, cubeb is cultivated for its fruit and essential oil.

Principal constituents: Contains sesquiterpenes, sesquiterpene alcohols and small amounts of monoterpenes.

Aromatherapy uses: It has natural antiseptic, antimicrobial and astringent properties useful for gum and teeth infections. It's used for digestive problems, controls flatulence and regulates bowel movements. It detoxifies the body. It also helps clear phlegm and eases respiration, and is also reputed to be an aphrodisiac.

Description and odour effect: The oil is colourless to light green with a spicy odour and acrid taste. It has calming properties and is used during stress and hypertension.

Caution: May cause skin irritation in some individuals. Do not use on facial skin and contact with eyes should be avoided.

CUMIN SEED
(Cuminum cyminum)
Family: Labiatae/Lamiaceae

Source: Originally from the Mediterranean area, cumin is a small annual herb about 50 centimetres high with narrow, deep green feathery leaves, tiny white or pink flowers, and small oblong seeds. In use for over 4000 years, cumin is mainly used in cooking. Today it is popular in the cuisines of India. The essential oil is extracted through steam distillation of the seeds.

Principal constituents: Cuminic aldehyde.

Aromatherapy use: Helps bloating, constipation, diarrhoea, gas, indigestion, heartburn, headache, and stomach pain. The oil helps to fight cancer, promotes liver health and helps control diabetes. It also helps weight loss.

Description and odour effect: A thin, pale yellow-greenish to brownish liquid with a middle note. It has a characteristic warm, spicy, musky aroma.

Caution: This essential oil has phototoxic properties and exposure to the sun must be avoided after application to the skin. Consult a physician prior to using this oil. Dilute well before use; for external use only. May cause skin irritation in some individuals. Contact with eyes should be avoided.

DILL
(Anethum graveolens)
Family: Umbelliferae/Apiaceae

Source: Steam distillation of the seeds.

Principal constituents: The oil has a high ketone content, mostly dextro-carvone and phenolic ethers.

Aromatherapy uses: Dill seed oil is used in gripe water for babies. It helps the flow of bile, thus aiding digestion, and is useful for catarrhal conditions like bronchitis. Can be used for external application or tisanes.

Caution: Because of its high ketone content, the oil should not be used on children or pregnant women.

ELEMI
(Canarium luzonicum)
Family: Burseraceae

Source: Steam distillation of the gum exuding from the tall tree native to the Philippines and the Moluccas.

Principal constituents: Phellandrene, dispentene, limonene and pinene.

Aromatherapy uses: Rheumatic conditions, respiratory disorders, skin infections, nervous exhaustion. Can be used for inhalation, vaporisation, massage and application.

Description and odour effect: A pale yellow or colourless liquid with a strong, spicy balasmic aroma, which also has a citrus-geranium note. The odour effect is tenacious, stimulating and warming.

Caution: Use in the lowest concentration as it has a high odour intensity. Solvent-extracted oil can also irritate the skin.

FENNEL SEED, SWEET
(Foeniculum vulgare)
Family: Umbelliferae/Apiaceae

Source: Steam distillation of the crushed seeds from the herb native to the Mediterranean region. Most of the oil is produced in Hungary, Bulgaria, Germany, France, Italy, India and Greece.

Principal constituents: Anethole up to 60%, anisic aldehyde, camphene, d-fenchone, dipentene.

Aromatherapy uses: Bruises, cellulite, fluid retention, constipation, loss of appetite, flatulence, insufficient milk in nursing mothers, menopausal problems. Also helps detoxify the body. Can be used in a massage mix or tisane.

Description and odour effect: A colourless to pale yellow liquid with a sweet anise-like aroma. The odour effect is warming and stimulating.

Caution: The oil may irritate the skin so should be used with caution. Avoid during pregnancy. The oil has an intense odour, so use in small quantities. There is also a remote chance that fennel will promote an epileptic seizure, but only in prone subjects. Therefore, avoid for people suffering from epilepsy.

FIR, BALSAM *(Abies balsamea)*
Family: Pinaceae

Source: Native to North America, balsam fir has needles about 19–32 millimetres long with two white stripes running down the underside of each needle. It is also known as blistering pine. The essential oil is extracted through steam distillation of the needles of the plant.

Principal constituents: a- and b-pinene. lso-bornyl acetate.

Aromatherapy uses: With an uplifting yet soothing effect, **balsam fir essential oil** is an excellent **oil** for calming muscles and joints after a long day or intense workout. When diffused or applied topically to the chest, this **oil** can help support a healthy respiratory system. The oil is also used in air fresheners and household cleansers.

FIR NEEDLE *(Abies siberica)*
Family: Pinaceae

Source: Fir needle comes from the **Siberian fir** that grows in wide areas of Russia. Scandinavians used fir needles in the sauna and it was used as an aromatic in bedding. Oil is extracted from the needles through steam distillation.

Principal constituents: a-pinene, limonene and B-phelandren, bornyl acetate.

Aromatherapy uses: Fir needle essential **oil** is used to fight sore throats and respiratory infections, fatigue, muscle aches and arthritis.

Description and odour effect: A medium, clear, colourless to pale yellow liquid, fir needle oil has a sharp crisp clean scent typical of fir.

Caution: Dilute very well before use; for external use only. May cause skin irritation in some individuals. Contact with eyes should be avoided.

GALBANUM *(Ferula galbaniflua)*
Family: Umbelliferae/Apiaceae

Source: Water or steam distillation of the gum exuded by the large herb native to the Middle East and Western Asia.

Principal constituents: 50–60% carvone, sesquiterpenes, sesquiterpenic alcohol (cadinol) and terpenes (limonene and pinene).

Aromatherapy uses: Abscesses, acne, scars, wounds, inflamed skin, poor circulation, muscular aches and pains, rheumatism, respiratory ailments, nervous tension and stress-related disorders. Used in massage or application. Galbanum oil is also commonly used in the perfume and fragrance industry.

Description and odour effect: An amber-coloured liquid, becoming viscous as it ages, with a green-woody scent and soft balsamic undertone. The odour effect is calming; a reputed aphrodisiac.

Caution: Not to be used during pregnancy. The oil has an intense odour, so use in a low concentration.

GARLIC *(Allium sativum)*
Family: Amaryllidaceae (sub-family Allioideae)

Source: Garlic was worshipped by the ancient Egyptians, chewed by Greek Olympian athletes, and in eastern Europe was thought to keep vampires at bay. The plant has been used over many centuries in different countries as a protection against evil. Oil is extracted from the bulb by steam distillation.

Principal constituents: Diisopropyl disulfide, Diisopropyl trisulfide, allicin.

Aromatherapy uses: Treats acne: garlic oil is an excellent remedy for bad skin. As garlic is full of antioxidants it helps to boost immunity. Massaging a drop on the teeth and gums relieves toothache. The compound allicin helps in minimising tooth pain and helping to control bacterial build-up.

Also helps prevent hair fall. However, the smell of the oil is so overpowering that it will take over the odour of other essential oils.

Description and odour effect: A thin, clear, yellow to orange liquid. A very strong and pungent aroma.

Caution: Dilute before use; for external use only. May cause skin irritation in some individuals. Contact with eyes should be avoided. Keep in an airtight metal or dark glass container in isolation.

GINGER *(Zingiber officinale)*
Family: Zingiberaceae

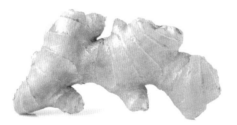

Source: Steam distillation of the unpeeled, dried, ground root (rhizomes) of the plant native to Southern Asia.

Principal constituents: Sesquiterpenes (camphene, d-phellandrene, zingiberene), sesquiterpenic alcohols (isoborneol-linalool) and terpenes.

Aromatherapy uses: Arthritis, muscular aches and pains, poor circulation, rheumatism, catarrh, coughs, sore throats, diarrhoea, colic, indigestion, nausea, travel sickness, colds and flu, debility, nervous exhaustion.

Description and odour effect: A pale yellow or amber liquid with a warm, peppery spicy scent, not as pleasantly pungent as the fresh root. Its odour effect is warming and stimulating; a reputed aphrodisiac.

Caution: Use in minute quantities as the intense aroma may overpower blends.

GRAPEFRUIT *(Citrus x paradisi)*
Family: Rutaceae

Source: Expression of the fresh peel of the fruit from the small evergreen tree native to tropical Asia. A low-grade oil with a less attractive odour is obtained by steam distillation of the peel and fruit pulp. The oil is mainly produced in California.

Principal constituents: Monoterpenes – limonene (96–98%), aldehydes, coumarins, furocoumarins.

Aromatherapy uses: Cellulite, muscle fatigue, fluid retention, chills, colds and flu, depression, nervous exhaustion.

Description and odour effect: The expressed oil (not the lower grade extraction) is a yellow-green liquid with a fresh, sweet citrus fragrance. Its odour effect is uplifting and antidepressant.

Caution: Do not apply to the skin shortly before exposure to sunlight as it may cause pigmentation.

HELICHRYSUM/IMMORTELLE
(Helichrysum italicum syn. H. angustifolia)
Family: Compositae/Asteraceae

Source: One of the rare oils today, helichrysum is extracted by steam distillation of the flowers of this Mediterranean plant.

Principal constituents: Sesquiterpenes – mainly B caryophyllene, monoterpenol – nerol, esters – neryl acetate (75%), and ketones – b diones (italidione i, ii, iii) up to 20%.

Aromatherapy uses: Helichrysum, or immortelle, was one of the oils used by Jesus for healing work. European researchers have found helichrysum an effective regenerator of tissues, nerves and circulation. The **oil** has anti-inflammatory, antioxidant, antimicrobial, antifungal and antibacterial properties. It is useful for all skin problems like acne, infections, burns, eczema, bruising, cuts and dermatitis. Also useful for the circulatory system; acts as detoxifier, decongestant and cleanser. Can be used for massage or application.

Description and odour effect: The oil has a soft pervading sweet but uplifting aroma, and helps to relieve anxiety, lethargy, tension, stress and shock.

Caution: The oil may be neuro sensitive due to the high ketone content.

HYSSOP *(Hysoppus officinalis)*
Family: Labiatae/Lamiaceae

Source: Steam distillation of the flowers of a hardy green plant with narrow dark leaves similar to those of lavender and rosemary.

Principal constituents: Alcohol, geraniol, borneol, thujone, phellandrene, and a terpenic ketone – pinocamphone – in large quantities.

Aromatherapy uses: Hyssop is pectoral, expectorant, decongestant, stimulant, sudorific and carminative. It is useful for coughs, flu, bronchitis, asthma and chronic catarrh. Hyssop can also be used externally and one of the recommendations is to use as a poultice of young bruised leaves on a bruise, cut or wound. Can also be used for inhaltion and vaporisation.

Description and odour effect: The plant is cultivated for its essential oil in different parts of France. This oil has a pleasant, very aromatic odour and is dark yellowish.

Caution: The oil is a potential neurotoxin because it contains pinocamphone, so should be used with extreme care. It should only be sold to health practitioners and be available by prescription only.

JASMINE *(Jasminum grandiflorum; J. sambac)*
Family: Oleaceae

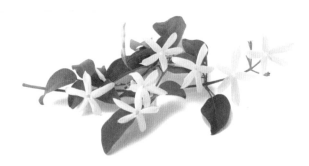

Source: Jasmine essential oil is as olvent-extracted from *J. grandiflorum* (chameli) and *J. sambac* (mogra). Both are night-scented evergreen climbers native to China, northern India and western Asia. Most of the oil is produced in Egypt and France. In India, both flowers are worn as *veni* (string) by women in their hair, for the sensual scent.

Principal constituents: Mainly jasmone, alpha terpineol, benzyl alcohol, indol, linalool and linalyl acetate.

Aromatherapy uses: A reputed antidepressant and aphrodisiac, also good for nervous exhaustion and stress-related conditions. Also helps balance the sacral (swadhisthan) chakra. It can be used for application, inhalation or vaporisation.

Description and odour effect: The absolute is dark amber and slightly viscous with a warm, floral scent and musky undertone. The fragrance improves as the oil ages. The odour of *J. grandiflorum* is pervading, sweet, sensuous and uplifting, while the fragrance of *J. sambac* is highly uplifting with a citrus touch.

Caution: The oil can be neuro sensitive due to its high ketone content.

JATAMANSI, INDIAN SPIKENARD
(Nardostachys jatamansi)
Family: Valerianaceae

Source: Jatamansi is distilled from the roots of a plant from India.

Principal constituents: Sesquiterpenes (93%), isobornyl valerianate, bornyl acetate, pinene, terpineol, eugenol, borneol, etc.

Aromatherapy uses: Reputed and regarded as a medicinal herb in India. It is antibacterial, antifungal and anti-inflammatory. Helps in the treatment of skin allergies, rashes, candida, flatulence, tension, migraine and insomnia. Can be used for vaporisation, application or massage.

Description and odour effect: The oil is amber-coloured, having a woody spicy, musty aroma. It has a sedating effect on the nervous system; helps in insomnia, nervous tension and migraines.

LAVANDIN *(Lavendula x intermedia)*
Family: Labiatae/Lamaceae

Source: Steam distillation of hybrid lavender, a cross between *L. angustifolia* and *L. latifolia*.

Principal constituents: Borneol (40–50%), camphor (10%), cineole (10%), geraniol, linalool and linayl acetate (15–35%).

Aromatherapy uses: The oil is mostly used in perfumery, but is also good for muscular, respiratory and circulatory problems because of its high camphor content. Used in massage or application.

Description and odour effect: The oil is yellow to dark yellow and smells acridly aromatic and a little camphoric.

Caution: Lavandin is less therapeutic than lavender but is often sold as lavender.

LEMONGRASS
(Cymbopogon citratus; C. flexuosus)
Family: Gramineae/Poaceae

Source: Steam distillation of leaves of tropical grasses native to tropical Asia and cultivated in India, Sri Lanka, Indonesia, Africa, Madagasscar, and North and South America. It resembles closely palmarosa and citronella, which are in the same genus.

Principal constituents: Citral (70–85%), dispentene, citronellal, farnesol, geraniol, limonene, linalool, myrcene, n-decyclic aldehyde, nerol.

Aromatherapy uses: A very uplifting mental stimulant. Very good antiseptic and detoxifying agent. Helps reduce temperature. Can be used in vaporisation or a massage mix.

Descrption and odour effect: A pale yellow liquid with citrus n-decyclic aldehyde top note, very good antidepressant and uplifting.

Caution: Due to the high citral content, the oil may sometimes cause skin irritation in people with sensitive skin. Do a patch test before using on skin.

LIME
(Citrus aurantifolia)
Family: Rutaceae

Source: Expression of the peel of the unripe fruit of the small evergreen tree native to southern Asia. There is also a distilled oil which is captured from the whole ripe crushed fruit. Most of the oil is produced in Florida, Cuba, Mexico and Italy.

Aromatherapy uses: Cellulite, poor circulation, respiratory disorders, colds and flu, depression. It is used for inhalation, vaporisation, application and massage.

Description and odour effect: A pale yellow or green liquid with a fresh, citrus aroma. Try to use within one year of purchase as the aroma rapidly deteriorates with age. The odour effect is uplifting and refreshing.

Caution: The expressed oil can cause unsightly blotching of the skin if applied shortly before exposure to sunlight, as the oil is photosensitive, but the distilled oil is benign in this respect. However, the aroma of the expressed oil is superior.

MANDARIN *(Citrus reticulata)*
Family: Rutaceae

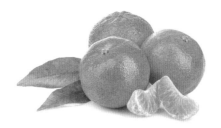

Source: Expression of the peel of the fruit of the small evergreen tree native to southern China and the Far East. Most of the oil is produced in Italy, Spain, Cyprus and Greece.

Principal constituents: Methyl anthranilate, limonene, geraniol and terpenic aldehydes.

Aromatherapy uses: A relaxing and uplifting oil which helps with stretch marks, cellulite, fluid retention, digestive problems, insomnia and nervous tension. Can be used in vaporisation and massage.

Description and odour effect: A yellow-orange liquid with an intensely sweet citrus aroma. Try to use within one year of purchase as the aroma rapidly deteriorates with age. The odour effect is soothing and uplifting.

Caution: Do not apply to the skin shortly before exposure to sunlight as it may cause pigmentation due to its photosensitive nature.

MAY CHANG *(Litsea cubeba)*
Family: Lauraceae

Source: *L. cubeba* is a small plant found in tropical areas. The leaves are green with a pleasant, lemony smell. It produces small, pepper-like fruits from which the essential oil is extracted by steam distillation. It has traditionally been used in Japan and Taiwan.

Principal constituents: Citral (up to 70%)

Aromatherapy uses: Controls high blood pressure. May chang oil has hypotensive properties. Prevents fungal infections and acts as a fungicide. Aids digestion: may chang oil has stomachic properties.

Description and odour effect: A thin, clear, pale yellow to yellow liquid with a top note and crisp, citrus smell. It can be compared to lemongrass and lemon verbena, but it is sweeter than lemongrass, without the musty note, and more accurately citrus in its scent than melissa.

Caution: For external use only. May cause skin irritation in some individuals. Contact with eyes should be avoided.

MELISSA *(Melissa officinalis)*
Family: Labiatae/Lamiaceae

Source: Steam distillation of the leaves and tops of a hardy herbaceous perennial native to southern Europe.

Principal constituents: Citral, citronellal, geraniol, linonene, linalool and pinene.

Aromatherapy uses: Clinical trials have shown melissa to be a good antidepressant, besides being antispasmodic, an emmanagogic, a stimulant for the nervous system and a tonic for the cardiac system, and good for headaches, anxiety, palpitations and insomnia. Used in vaporisation, inhalation and massage.

Description and odour effect: Oil is pale yellow with an agreeable and subtle, warm, lemony aroma, which is pleasantly uplifting.

MYRRH
(Commiphora myrrha)
Family: Burseraceae

Source: Steam distillation of the gum of the small tree native to north-east Africa and south-west Asia. A solvent-extracted resinoid is also available, but this is not recommended as it is solid at room temperature and therefore difficult to use.

Principal constituents: Acids (acetic, formic, myrrholic, palmitic, triterpenic etc.), alcohols, aldehydes (cinnamic, cuminic etc.), sugars (arabinose, galactose, etc.), phenols (eugenol, m-cresol), resins, and terpenes (cadinene, dipentene, limonene, pinene, etc).

Aromatherapy uses: Athlete's foot, skincare (especially mature skins), ringworm, wounds, arthritis, respiratory disorders, gum infections, mouth ulcers, absence of menstruation outside pregnancy, thrush, nervous tension. Used in vaporisation, inhalation and massage.

Description and odour effects: The essential oil is a light amber viscous liquid with a warm balsamic odour, which improves as the oil ages. Its odour effect is warming and relaxing.

Caution: Not to be used during pregnancy.

MYRTLE *(Myrtus communis)*
Family: Myrtaceae

Source: Steam distillation of the fresh leaves of an evergreen shrub which originates in Africa and grows all around the Mediterranean.

Principal constituents: The oil contains a lot of tannin, camphene, cineole, geraniol, linalool, pinene and myrtenol.

Aromatherapy uses: The oil is a tonic and astringent, used in skin preparations. Also effective against haemorrhoids, due to its high tannic content. Used in application and massage.

Description and odour effects: The oil is clear yellow to greenish yellow. It smells camphory and peppery green, rather like bay.

NIAOULI *(Melaleuca viridiflora)*
Family: Myrtaceae

Source: Steam distillation of the fresh leaves and twigs of an evergreen tree growing principally in New Caledonia and Australia.

Principal constituents: Eucalyptol (50–60%) plus a few esters (butyric and isovalerianic), limonene, pinene and terpineol.

Aromatherapy uses: Strong antiseptic, prescribed mainly for the urinary system (cystitis and leucorrhoea) and pulmonary trouble (bronchitis, catarrh, runny or stuffy nose). Use in sitz bath, compress, vaporisation, inhalation and massage.

Description and odour effect: The oil is a pale yellow that can become dark yellow (depending on the copper content of the soil). It has a strong hot smell, very balsamic with a note of camphor. It is similar to cajuput in aroma and therapeutic properties.

Caution: Sometimes the oil can cause skin irritation in people with sensitive skin.

NUTMEG *(Myristica fragrans)*
Family: Myristicaceae

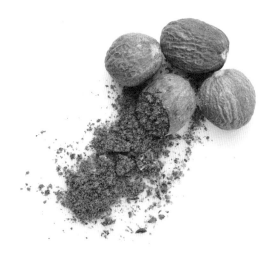

Source: Trees that produce both nutmeg and mace are large evergreens native to the Moluccas. Nutmeg oil is steam-distilled from nuts, crushed to a butter. The oil imported from the islands, is redistilled in France to improve the quality. Mace is steam-distilled from the arils (seed coverings).

Principal constituents: Both oils contain myristicin, with small quantities of sabinene, beta pinene, limonene, gamma terpinene, terpinen-4-ol, elmicin, beta-phellandrene and alpha thujene.

Aromatherapy uses: In the eighteenth century, in France, mace was classified as a tonic and stimulant, as an aid for general fatigue, and as a brain stimulant. It is also revered for its digestive properties, for people who cannot assimilate food, for wind, and for premenstrual pain. Nutmeg too is a tonic, good for the heart and for convalescence. Nutmeg also has a reputation as an abortifacient. Used in inhalation and massage.

Description and odour effect: Both oils are similar, very pale yellow and very fluid. Nutmeg smells spicy, pleasant and hot; mace very strongly spicy. Both oils change as they become old, turning dark brown and smelling disagreeably acidic and turpentine like, hence should not be used.

Caution: Myristicin is narcotic, hallucinogenic and very toxic, especially during pregnancy. Nutmeg mace oil should be avoided or used with great caution. It is better to use the spice instead of the oil for its therapeutic benefits.

OAKMOSS *(Evernia prunastri)*
Family: Parmeliaceae

Source: Solvent extraction of a lichen found growing on oak trees and sometimes on other species. The lichen is indigenous to Europe and North America.

Aromatherapy uses: Not generally used in aromatherapy, though the oil is said to be antiseptic, demulcent (protects mucous membranes and allays irritation) and expectorant. Can be used in vaporisation and inhalation.

Decription and odour effect: A dark green, viscous liquid with an extremely tenacious earthy-mossy odour. The odour improves as the oil ages. Its effect is warming and calming.

ORANGE, SWEET *(Citrus x sinensis)*
Family: Rutaceae

Source: Expression of the fresh ripe peel of the fruit of the small evergreen tree native to the Far East. An inferior-grade steam-distilled oil, obtained from the fruit pulp, is also available. Most of the oil is produced in Italy, Tunisia, Morocco and France.

Principal constituents: Up to 90% limonene with aldehydes, citral, citronellol, geraniol, linalool, methyl anthranilate, nonyl alcohol and terpineol.

Aromatherapy uses: Palpitations, fluid retention, respiratory ailments, colds and flu, nervous tension, stress and depression. Used in inhalation, vaporisation and massage.

Description and odour effect: A pale yellow liquid with a warm, sweet citrus scent. Try to use within one year of purchase as the aroma rapidly deteriorates with age. Its odour effect is uplifting.

Caution: Do not apply to the skin shortly before exposure to sunlight as it may cause pigmentation.

OREGANO *(Origanum vulgare)*
Family: Labiatae/Lamiaceae

Source: Steam-distilled from the leaves and flowers of the plant from the mint family, mainly from Utah, Turkey and France.

Principal constituents: Monoterpenes (25%) – alpha and beta pinene, myrcene, sequiterpene, monoterpenols, linalool and phenols (60–72%), carvacrol, thymol.

Aromatherapy uses: Powerfully anti-infectious with a large spectrum against bacteria, fungus and parasites for the respiratory system, intestines, genitals, nerves, blood and lymphatics. The oil also helps in urinary infections, nephritis, digestive problems and balances metabolism. Can also be used on skin warts. Used in application in dilution.

Description and odour effect: An amber-yellow liquid with a warm, pungent aroma, helps control fainting.

Caution: A very strong oil. Do not apply to skin directly. Always use in dilution.

PALO SANTO *(Bursera graveolens)*
Family: Burseraceae

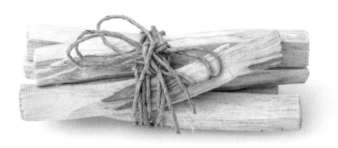

Source: Palo santo is found originally in tropical forests on the coast of the South Pacific, but Ecuador is now the main country where this tree is harvested. Palo santo oil is found only in the interior of the tree's trunk. It can take up to 10 years to produce the oil, which is steam-distilled from the wood of the plant. The Ecuadorans used it to perfume their homes. It was also used in rituals by shamans.

Principal constituents: Limonene.

Aromatherapy uses: Palo santo benefits immune health and inflammation. Palo santo oil has been found to contain cancer-fighting compounds that lower oxidative stress and protect cells. Its protective phytochemicals seem capable of helping to stop disease formation within the digestive, endocrine, cardiovascular and nervous systems.

Description and odour effect: A top note with a medium aroma, palo santo essential oil has a fresh, intense woody aroma with a slight hint of citrus. It is a thin, clear, pale yellow to light brown liquid.

Caution: Dilute well before use; for external use only. May cause skin irritation in some individuals. Contact with eyes should be avoided.

PETITGRAIN *(Citrus aurantium* var. *amara)*
Family: Rutaceae

Source: Steam distillation of the leaves and twigs of the bitter orange tree native to southern China and north-east India. Most of the oil is produced in France.

Principal constituents: Geraniol and geranyl acetate, limonene, linalool, linalyl acetate and sesquiterpene.

Aromatherapy uses: Astringent, good for oily skin conditions, nervous exhaustion and stress-related disorders. Used in vaporisation, inhalation, application and massage.

Description and odour effect: A pale yellow liquid with a fresh, woody, bittersweet scent reminiscent of neroli, but less refined. Its odour effect is refreshing and uplifting.

PINE, SCOTCH *(Pinus sylvestris)*
Family: Pinaceae

Source: Dry distillation of the needles of the evergreen tree native to Scotland and Norway. Most of the oil is produced in the eastern USA from cultivated trees.

Principal constituents: Borneol acetate 30–40% (which is what differentiates it from turpentine). Other terpenes are cadinene, dispentene and phellandrene, pinene and sylvesterene.

Aromatherapy uses: Astringent. Controls excessive perspiration, arthritis, muscular aches and pains, poor circulation, rheumatism, respiratory ailments, cystitis, colds and flu, fatigue and nervous exhaustion.

Description and odour effect: A colourless to pale yellow liquid with a dry-balsamic, turpentine-like aroma.

Its odour effect is cooling and mentally stimulating, yet also comforting to the emotions.

Caution: Avoid going out in sun after using the oil as may cause skin irritation.

RAVENSARA *(Ravensara aromatica)*
Family: Lauraceae

Source: Steam-distilled from the branches of a plant of the laurel family from Madagascar.

Principal constituents: Monoterpenes alpha and beta pinene, sesquiterpenes, monoterpenols, terpinic esters and oxides 1–8 cineole.

Aromatherapy uses: Excessive perspiration, arthritis, muscular aches and pains, poor circulation, rheumatism, respiratory ailments, cystitis, colds and flu, fatigue, nervous exhaustion. Described as 'the oil that heals' in Madagascar, it is found to be anti-infectious, antibacterial, antiviral, antimicrobial and expectorant. It is a tonic for the nerves and the respiratory system, and effective for bronchitis and respiratory infections. Useful in the treatment of herpes simplex and herpes zoster. Also helps in childhood viral infections like chicken pox and measles. Used in gargles, inhalation, application and massage.

Description and odour effect: A colourless to pale yellow liquid helpful for fatigue, burnout and tension.

ROSEWOOD *(Aniba rosaeodora)*
Family: Lauraceae

Source: Steam-distilled from the wood of a plant of the laurel family from Brazil.

Principal constituents: Monoterpenols, mainly linalool (85–95%), little oxides, monoterpenes and sequiterpenes.

Aromatherapy uses: Due to its high alcoholic percentage, the oil is effective and safe for skincare, good for bacterial infections, urinary, bronchial, ear, nose and throat infections, and skin conditions like dermatitis. Used in gargles, vaporisation, application and massage.

Description and odour effect: A pale yellow liquid with sweet wood aroma that helps to relieve mental and physical exhaustion; relieves depression.

SAGE
(Salvia officinalis)
Family: Labiatae/Lamiaceae

Source: Steam distillation of the flowers and leaves of a hardy, evergreen shrub native to southern Europe.

Principal constituents: Borneol, camphor, cineole, alpha-pinene, salvene and thujone (22–61%).

Aromatherapy uses: Sage has been cultivated for centuries for its culinary and medicinal properties. It helps in several skin conditions such as eczema, alopecia and ulcers. Helps in rheumatic and general aches and pains. Alleviates low blood pressure, purifies blood, regulates menstrual flow; a good diuretic and beneficial in menopause. The oil is also used to cleanse the auric field. Used in vaporisation, inhalation and massage.

Description and odour effect: The oil is colourless to pale yellow with a strong herbaceous smell.

Caution: Due to its thujone content, the oil can stimulate the nervous system and can cause epileptic fits in prone subjects – use with care.

SAVORY, SUMMER *(Satureja hortensis)*; SAVORY, WINTER *(S. montana)*
Family: Labiatae/Lamiaceae

Source: Steam distillation is performed on the leaves (and sometimes flowers) of two major savory varieties: summer savory – an annual growing to 30–60 centimetres high with dark green aromatic leaves, hairy stems and lilac-pink flowers; and winter savory, which is compact and erect with small grey-green leaves and tiny rose-purple flowers. Both are plants of the Mediterranean region.

Principal constituents: The oil has a very high phenol content. Other constituents are 30–40% carvacrol, 20–30% thymol and cineole, cymene amd pinene.

Aromatherapy uses: The oil is strongly antiseptic because of its high phenol content, so should be used in dilution. Very useful for hastening the formation of scar tissue and for treating bites, burns, ulcers and abscesses. Used in application and massage. Herb tea with fresh savory is a great tonic; wine with savory is an aphrodisiac.

Description and odour effect: The oil is pale orange, quite hot, like thyme, and a bit acrid.

Caution: May irritate the skin. Do a patch test before using.

SPEARMINT *(Mentha spicata)*
Family: Labiatae/Lamiaceae

Source: The oil is produced by steam distillation of the leaves of an evergreen plant of the mint family.

Principal constituents: Borneol monoterpenes – limonene, pinene, myrcene, etc, along with monoterpenols – menthol, linalool, and ketones (55–65%) – carvone, dihydrocarvone and menthone.

Aromatherapy uses: Digestive oil, so good for acidity, heartburn, intestinal parasites and bad breath; also helps in hot flushes, nausea, nervousness, headaches and migraines. Used in tisanes, gargles, inhalation, vaporisation and application.

Description and odour effect: A greenish-yellow liquid with a strong minty aroma commonly used for chewing gums, candies and toiletries.

Caution: Be careful when using on skin as the oil is strong and may irritate.

SPRUCE
(Picea mariana)
Family: Pinaceae

Source: The black spruce is a tree native to Canada. It is typically found in wet, swampy areas where the wild trees can grow up to 15 metres in height. The oil is extracted from the needles and twigs through steam distillation.

Principal constituents: a-pinene, bornyl acetate.

Aromatherapy uses: Provides emotional healing. **Spruce essential oil** is both stimulating and calming. It improves concentration, focus, and memory and provides relaxation from mental stresses.

Description and odour effect: Colourless to pale yellow liquid with a top note. It is sweeter and softer than most evergreen oils with a balsamic, resinous odour with green woody notes. Overall, the scent is very clean, fresh and pleasant.

Caution: Black spruce essential oil should be applied to the skin only in dilution as it has the potential to irritate. Avoid use during pregnancy.

STAR ANISE *(Illicium verum)*
Family: Schisandraceae

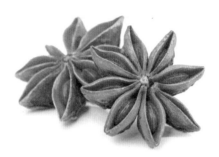

Source: Star anise is a smaller plant belonging to the magnolia family, native to China and Vietnam, although today it is grown almost exclusively in southwest China and Japan. The fruit is small, only about 3 centimetres long and star-shaped with 5–10 points. The fruit is picked unripe and sun-dried before it is used. The oil is extracted from seeds by steam distillation.

Principal constituents: T-anethole (86–96%).

Aromatherapy uses: Used to promote peaceful sleep, relieve indigestion and intestinal issues and ease breathing. Also a natural remedy for PMS symptoms. Useful to soothe intestines and reduce flatulence.

Description and odour effect: A thin, colourless to pale yellow liquid with a top note and strong aroma. Star anise has a scent similar to licorice and aniseed, but stronger.

Caution: Dilute before use; for external use only. May cause skin irritation in some individuals; a skin test is recommended prior to use. Contact with eyes should be avoided.

Note: This oil may form crystals during transit or storage. Gentle warming in a hot water bath and stirring may be required.

TAGETES *(Tagetes minuta* syn. *T. glandulifera)*
Family: Compositae/Asteraceae

Source: Steam distillation of the flowers of the African marigold plant, sometimes confused with calendula.

Aromatherapy uses: Effective on slow-to-heal wounds, burns and bruises, it is also useful against catarrhal conditions. Competent on fungal infections of the feet and of the digestive system (candida). May also promote the onset of menstruation. It is an excellent deterrent to house flies. Can be used in vaporisation and application.

Principal constituents: Contains approximately 35–50% tagetone, a ketone, and its coumarin content makes it a photosensitiser. Can be used in vaporisation and application.

Caution: Dilute well before use. Being neurotoxic it should only be used by experienced aromatherapists. Not recommended for use on pregnant women or on children. Do not use immediately before exposure to sun. May cause skin irritation in some individuals.

TANSY, BLUE
(Tanacetum annuum L.)
Family: Asteraceae/Compositae

Source: Blue tansy is also known as true Moroccan chamomile. Another species grown in Morocco, *Ormensis multicaulis*, is correctly called wild Moroccan chamomile, but it does not have the distinctive blue colour of the other chamomiles. Blue tansy, like other blue essential oils, contains the active azulene. The oil is steam-distilled from the leaves and flowers.

Principal constituents: Sabinene, chamazulene (**up to 5%**).

Aromatherapy uses: Blue tansy essential oil has both antibacterial and antifungal properties. Blue tansy also has potent antihistamine and anti-inflammatory properties hence also good for allergies and muscle relief and arthritis. Blue tansy essential oil has a delightful warm, herbaceous aroma that can relieve anxiety and stress.

Description and odour effect: A thick, blue liquid with a middle note, blue tansy has a surprisingly sweet aroma.

Caution: Dilute before use; for external use only. May cause skin irritation in some individuals.

TARRAGON
(Artemisia dracunculus)
Family: Asteraceae/Compositae

Source: Tarragon is a perennial herb that thrives near water. It has a woody stem that reaches to about 1 metre tall. The leaves are silver-green and covered with fine silky hairs, and the flowers are pale yellow. The name is derived from the Arabic word *tharkhoum* and the Latin word *dracunculus*, meaning 'little dragon' probably because of the way the root coils. Oil is extracted from the leaves through steam distillation.

Principal constituents: Methyl chavicol (78.2%).

Aromatherapy uses: Essential **oil** of **tarragon** improves the circulation of blood and lymph. Furthermore, it does not let **toxins** accumulate in particular places, such as the joints. Both the herb itself and the essential oil are known to help improve digestion.

Description and odour effect: A thin, clear, colourless to pale yellow liquid. A middle note with a medium aroma, tarragon essential oil has a richly sweet, anise-like green scent with spicy notes.

Caution: Dilute before use as it can be moderately toxic due to the methyl chavicol in the oil. May cause skin irritation in some individuals.

TURMERIC
(Curcuma longa)
Family: Zingiberaceae

Source: Turmeric is a perennial plant with roots or tubers. Typically grown in India, it is a deep orange on the inside and has roots about 2 feet long. Oil is extracted from the roots through steam distillation.

Main constituents: Turmerones (10–40%), alpha curcumin.

Aromatherapy uses: It has been in very wide use by women for skin care, and well known globally as a cooking spice. Lowers inflammation. Stimulates circulation. Turmeric oil is known as a stimulant, as it not only boosts metabolism and heart health, it has anticancer potential. Significant research has been conducted on both turmeric and turmeric oil, and the anti-mutagenic properties of this oil are well known.

Description and odour effect: Pale yellow to orange-yellow liquid. It has a base note with a medium aroma. The oil has the same fragrant woody scent as the powdered spice used in Eastern cuisine.

Caution: Dilute before use; for external use only. May cause skin irritation in some individuals; a skin test is recommended prior to use. Contact with eyes should be avoided.

VALERIAN *(Valeriana officinalis)*;
INDIAN VALERIAN *(V. wallichii)*
Family: Caprifoliaceae

Source: Steam distillation of the fresh, well-dried roots.

Principal constituents: The chemical constituent responsible for the aroma and therapeutic effect is bornyl-isovalerate, which develops as the roots are dried.

Aromatherapy uses: It is used almost exclusively for its powerfully calming effect on the nervous system, thus aiding all conditions related to severe mental stress, for example, insomnia, agitation, nervous headaches, nervous stomach, palpitations, etc. Best to use in inhalation or vaporisation. Can also be used for application.

Description and odour effect: Used as the blueprint for valium, the well-known sedative drug, valerian is known in aromatherapy for its rather pungent aroma. The aroma of Indian valerian (*V. wallichii*) is considered inferior; being strong, the oil is yellowy-brown in colour.

European valerian oil (*V. officinalis*) is blue-green depending on the amount of azulene produced during distillation.

Caution: Use over a long period may cause lethargy. Use only one drop in addition to petitgrain, orange or mandarin to improve the aroma.

YARROW, BLUE
(Achillea millefolium)
Family: Asteraceae/Compositae

Source: Yarrow is also known as milfoil, a reference to its feathery appearance from the fern-like leaves. It is a perennial herb with a simple stem that can grow up to one metre in height, bearing numerous pale pink flower heads. Yarrow has a long history as a medicinal herb, which goes back to the legend of Achilles, who used it for wounds inflicted during the Trojan War. Oil is steam distilled from the flowers.

Main constituents: Beta-pinene, sabinene, camphor.

Aromatherapy uses: Yarrow essential oil can be used to stem the blood oozing out of a wound. Yarrow essential oil is a remedy for varicose veins and hemorrhoids, and relieves arthritis pain. It is often used in cosmetics for dry skin.

Description and odour effect: A thin, clear, greenish to dark blue liquid. A top note with a medium aroma, yarrow is sweet and herbaceous, with spicy tones.

Caution: Dilute before use; for external use only. May cause skin irritation in some individuals; a skin test is recommended.

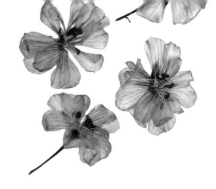

CARRIERS AND CARRIER OILS USED IN AROMATHERAPY

A 'carrier' carries the essential oil in an application. All essential oil applications require a carrier, although not necessarily an oil. We use various carriers, knowingly or unknowingly. Even in the simple process of inhalation, the air acts as a carrier; in a bath, sitz bath or douche it is water which acts as a carrier. Only a few essential oils can be used undiluted as they are highly concentrated and may sensitise the skin if used neat. Therefore it is recommended to dilute essential oils in fatty/ vegetable oils before we use them on the skin. Sometimes creams, lotions or gels are used as carriers.

CARRIER OR BASE OILS

Most preferred aromatherapy bases, or carriers, for skin application are cold-pressed vegetable oils as they enter easily through the skin pores so facilitate the penetration of essential oil into the body. Vegetable oils are also beneficial in other ways, acting as a balancing and stabilising agent as well as containing the minerals iodine, vitamin E and essential fatty acids (EFAs). EFAs are needed by the body as a part of our regular dietary intake.

They include oleic acid, linoleic acid and linolenic acid.

Fatty acids are of two types: saturated and unsaturated. The oils rich in saturated fatty acids are generally too thick and greasy so are not preferred for aromatherapy use. The unsaturated fatty acids are classified into two groups: monounsaturated and polyunsaturated. Fatty oils consisting primarily of oleic acid are called monounsaturated oils ('mono' meaning 'one'), as this fatty acid has only one double bond in its chemistry. The higher the proportion of oleic acid, the more stable the oil and it oxidises much more slowly, so monounsaturated oils such as almond, apricot, olive, hazelnut and camellia keep well for long time.

When a fatty oil contains a large amount of linoleic and linolenic fatty acids, the oil is known as a polyunsaturated oil ('poly' meaning 'many'), as these have two or three double bonds respectively. Examples include sunflower, soybean and wheatgerm. Polyunsaturated oils are light, not too greasy, but tend to break down easily, so therefore prone to oxidisation. Oils rich in polyunsaturated fatty acids are good for the heart, but in aromatherapy we need to choose a fatty oil that will not oxidise too readily. Oxidised fatty oils have free radicals, which are dangerous to the cells of the body. When a massage oil (consisting of essential oils in a fatty oil base) becomes rancid or oxidised, a chemical change takes place. This not only affects the fragrance of the blend and prevents the essential oils from working properly, but if massaged into the skin can introduce cell-damaging free radicals, causing skin irritation. Therefore choosing a correct carrier or base oil is as important as choosing the correct essential oils.

THE THREE CATEGORIES OF CARRIER OILS

Basic carrier oils: These form the highest proportion (40–60%) of an aromatherapy formulation, since they are easily available or low in price, etc. They include grapeseed oil, sesame oil and olive oil.

Specialised fixed oils: These are more often used as a certain percentage (10–30%) in a mixture; they may be too thick or too expensive to be used on their own. They render specific therapeutic or nourishing and moisturising properties to the whole mix. Examples include jojoba, avacado, rosehip, wheatgerm, evening primrose and hazelnut.

Macerated oils: These are plant extracts in a basic fixed oil. There are a few plants which contain very interesting properties, but whose essential oils are too difficult or too expensive to distil. In order to benefit from these properties, the plant materials are chopped up and put into a vat containing vegetable oil or water; this process is called maceration. The vegetable oil acts as a solvent, drawing essential oil from the plant material, including the small molecules as well as larger molecules such as plant colouring. The resulting liquid is then filtered and bottled. Macerated oils include calendula, carrot, hypericum, lime blossom and melissa.

Following is a chart of fatty oils, listing the oleic, linoleic and linolenic acid composition of each. The chart should be used as a guide to choose the best oil for your formulations, within constraints such as availability of the oil and the limitations of your budget.

COMPOSITION OF FATTY OILS					
	Classification	% Oleic	% Linoleic	% Linolenic	
Almond (sweet)	M	70	20	N/A	N
Apricot	M/P	65	27	N/A	N
Argan nut	M	43	37	<0.5	N
Avocado	M	70	9	N/A	N
Camellia	M	78–92	1–2.2	N/A	N
Coconut	Sat	6.5	1.5	N/A	N/A
Corn	P	19–49	34–62	1–2.7	S
Cotton seed	P	15.3–36	35–54.8	N/A	S
Grapeseed	P	14	74	N/A	S
Hazelnut	M	77	10	N/A	N
Jojoba – liquid wax	N/A	N/A	N/A	N/A	N
Olive	M	65–85	3.9–15	0–1	N
Peach kernel	M/P	68	25	N/A	N
Peanut	M	42.3–61.1	13–33.4	N/A	N
Pumpkin	P	35	45	N/A	S
Rice	P	40–50	29–42	0–1	S
Rosehip seed	P	15	47	28–30	N
Safflower	P	13	75	N/A	S
Sesame	M	35–46	35.2–48.4	0.2	N
Soybean	P	32.5–30.8	49.2–52	1.9–10	D
Sunflower	P	33	52	0–1	S

Key

M – Monounsaturated

P – Polyunsaturated

M/P – Borderline between M and P

Sat – Saturated

N – Non-drying

S – Semi-drying

D – Drying

N/A – Not available

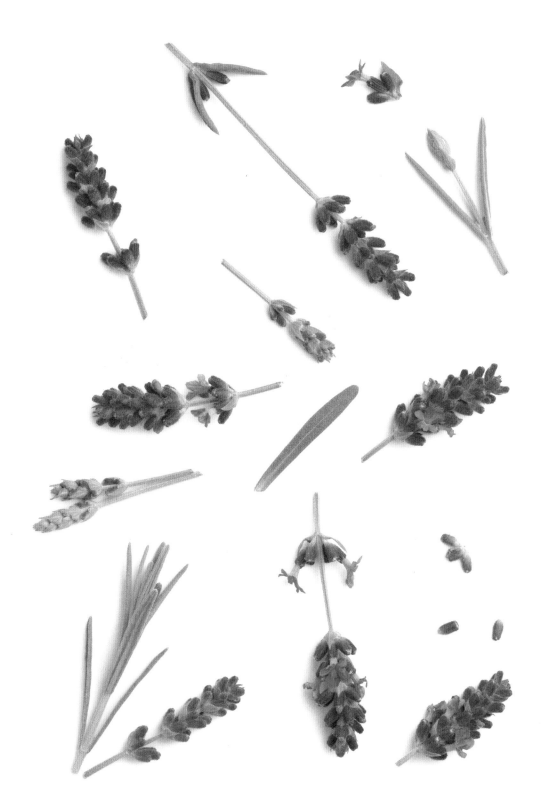

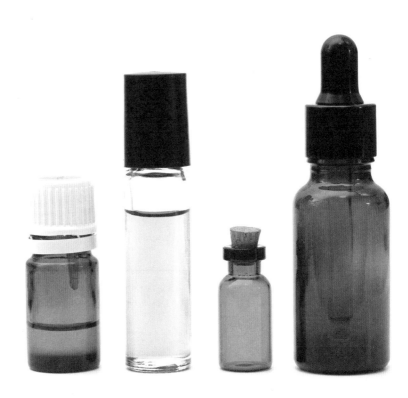

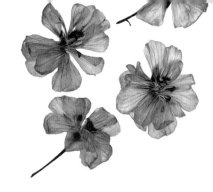

CARRIER OILS USED IN AROMATHERAPY

ALMOND OIL, SWEET *(Prunus amygdalus* var. *dulcis)*

The sweet almond tree yields a fixed oil obtained by cold-pressing.

Note: While there is an essential oil made from bitter almonds, it should not be used in aromatherapy because of the risk of prussic acid forming during distillation.

Properties and effects: Sweet almond oil contains vitamins A, B1, B2 and B6 and has a high percentage of mono- and polyunsaturated fatty acids. Its high percentage of monounsaturated fatty acids means it keeps reasonably well. Because it has a small amount of vitamin E, it protects and nourishes the skin and calms the irritation caused by eczema.

APRICOT KERNEL OIL *(Prunus armenica)*

Apricot, peach and sweet almond yield almost the same oils chemically (therefore having similar effects). Apricot and peach are usually more expensive as they are not produced in such great quantity. Occasionally, almond oil is sold as apricot or peach, so be sure of the source of your oil.

Properties and effects: One of the great advantages of this oil is that it is suitable for all skin types – dry, oily or mature. Apricot oil has soothing effects that heal burnings or irritations that may be on the face, either caused by the sun or allergic reactions. It also helps reduce inflammation and is good for massages for arthritis and gout.

ARGAN NUT OIL *(Argania spinosa)*

Argan trees grow and tenaciously survive in semi-desert areas of the Mediterranean. Argan oil is derived from the nuts of *A. spinosa*. The oil is rich in vitamins A and E, minerals, antioxidants and essential fatty acids as it is high in both oleic and linoleic acids. Pure argan nut oil is great to moisturise dry skin and damaged hair. Argan oil's high linoleic acid content helps to reduce inflammation caused by acne, while helping to soothe damaged skin cells. However, if you have a nut allergy, avoid using this oil. **Properties and effects**: Pure argan nut oil is great to moisturise dry skin and damaged hair. Argan oil's high linoleic acid content helps to reduce inflammation caused by acne, while helping to soothe damaged skin cells. However, if you have a nut allergy, avoid using this oil.

AVOCADO OIL *(Persea americana)*

Avocado oil is pressed from the dried and sliced flesh of fruits which are not good enough for sale as fresh produce. Being quite a difficult oil to press, it sometimes has a cloudy appearance – even a bit sludgy at the bottom. This should be regarded as a good sign and not a fault.

Avocado oil has excellent keeping qualities because of an inbuilt antioxidant system. However if chilled (or during the winter), some components are precipitated, causing it to go cloudy. This can be rectified by placing the bottle in a warm place, when the oil will soon return unharmed to normal.

Properties and effects: Avocado contains both saturated and monounsaturated fatty acids, vitamins A, B and D, and is rich in lecithin. It is thought that despite its viscosity, avocado has the ability to penetrate the upper layers of the skin. It is a good moisturiser for the skin.

Avocado is valuable to aromatherapists for its beneficial effect on dry skin and wrinkles, and it can form up to 25% of the total mix. Because of its emollient properties, it is sometimes used in sun preparations.

CALENDULA OIL – MACERATED *(Calendula officinalis)*

Although sold as a fixed oil, the calendula grown in Europe for medical purposes does not produce any fixed oil itself. The flowerheads contain too little essential oil to make distillation commercially viable, so all active therapeutic properties are extracted by maceration.

Properties and effects: Calendula oil has anti-inflammatory, antispasmodic, choleretic (increasing bile production) and vulnerary (helping to heal wounds) properties, rendering it effective on bedsores, broken veins, bruises, gum inflammations (and tooth extraction cavities), persistent ulcers, stubborn wounds and varicose veins. It is extremely effective on skin problems, rashes and, in particular, chapped and cracked skin, which makes it an excellent base oil to use when treating dry eczema.

Note: Hypericum and calendula make an excellent synergistic mix to which essential oils can be added. Although extremely beneficial on its own, the effects are enhanced when essential oils for the condition being treated are added to it. If adding 25 per cent or less to a basic carrier oil, the addition of the extra essential oils becomes more important.

CAMELLIA *(Camellia japonica)*

Camellia oil, as its full name suggests, comes from Japan. It is extracted from the seeds of an evergreen tree from the Theaceae family, primarily cultivated on the islands of Izu and Kyushu in Japan. Its Japanese name is 'tsubaki' oil and it is used in exclusive restaurants for cooking tempura vegetables and prawns dipped in butter before quick frying, as the oil is very stable at high temperature.

Properties and effects: The oil is virtually odourless with a very good keeping quality, having a long lifespan as very slow to oxidise as long as the bottle is kept tightly closed and out of sunlight. The oil is fairly thick but not so greasy, with an excellent skin-penetrating ability. In beauty care, the stability of camellia oil makes it a very useful fatty oil for facial and body use, as the dangers of rancidity and resultant free radicals are negligible. The skin-penetrating properties of camellia oil enhance the speed at which diluted essential oil reach the deeper levels of the skin.

CARROT OIL – MACERATED *(Daucus carota* subsp. *sativus)*

True fixed oil of carrot is extracted by maceration of the finely chopped traditional orange carrot roots in a vegetable oil such as soya or sunflower and is rich in betacarotene. It is called 'true' fixed oil of carrot, because there is an oil used extensively in the cosmetic industry called 'Carrot oil' that has never seen a carrot: the African marigold (tagetes) is also rich in betacarotene and this is sold as 'carrot' oil. It has similar properties to true carrot, but the oil is extremely concentrated with a deeper colour. It is not suitable for aromatherapy treatments.

Properties and effects: True carrot oil is rich in betacarotene, vitamins B, C, D and E, and essential fatty acids.

Useful on burns, carrot oil is anti-inflammatory. It is known to be an effective rejuvenator, delaying the ageing process with repeated use. It is therefore a useful ingredient in skin creams or oils that are used every day.

Caution: There are no contraindications for the use of true carrot oil, but excessive ingestion of carrots themselves, or their juice, can cause hypervitaminosis (the palms of the hands and soles of the feet become orange and the body skin dry and flaky, taking on an orange, suntanned look). If these symptoms are ignored, the whole system becomes toxic, causing death in extreme cases.

CASTOR OIL *(Ricinus communis)*

Castor oil comes from a tall, quick-growing perennial woody shrub or small tree. Native to India, it is now seen in many warm-climate countries. It is often grown as an ornamental, but is also of value as a windbreak and shade tree. It bears seed profusely, and it is these that are pressed for the oil. Castor oil was known to the Greeks and Romans as purgative or laxative, which is still the major role of the oil today; many common laxatives contain a proportion of castor oil.

Properties and effects: It has a very viscid consistency, is colourless, has a slight fragrance and is disagreeable to the taste. The major constituents are palmitic and other fatty acids, ricinoleic acid and glycerine.

The ancient Egyptians called the oil 'kiki', using it as an unguent for skin rashes, and in embalming. It is still useful for numerous skin complaints, ranging from eczema to dryness of the skin. For very dry eczema, mix 2 tablespoons of castor oil with 1 tablespoon of almond oil and 2 drops of wheatgerm oil and apply gently to the affected part. Because the oil is so viscid, it is a good idea to mix it with a light carrier oil to help penetration.

COCONUT OIL *(Cocos nucifera)*

Coconut oil does not occur naturally. The white flesh when pressed yields an odorous solid fat, which contains therapeutic properties. To obtain coconut oil, the fat is subjected to heat (as in hot extraction) and the top liquid fraction removed. This is usually deodorised for use in both the food and cosmetic industries, as its natural odour is overpowering even with the addition of essential oils. Being a fractionated oil, its use in aromatherapy, where we insist on everything being complete and whole, must be questioned, hence not recommended.

Properties and effects: Coconut oil is an emollient on hair and skin, and is reputed to help filter the sun's rays; however, on some people it can cause a rash, perhaps because it is not a complete product.

CORN OIL *(Zea mays)*

This oil is produced exclusively by hot extraction (the corn germ containing very little oil). Though a very light oil, it is not one of the preferred oils for aromatherapy.

EVENING PRIMROSE OIL *(Oenothera biennis)*

Rich in linoleic acid, a polyunsaturated fatty acid and containing a small percentage of gamma linoleic acid (GLA, said to reduce blood cholesterol), evening primrose oil is extremely useful for the prevention of heart disease. These essential fatty acids are vital for cell and body function and cannot be made by the body itself.

Properties and effects: Taken internally, evening primrose oil is said to be invaluable for reducing blood pressure, controlling arthritis, relieving eczema, helping schizophrenia, fibrocystic breast condition and PMS, and decreasing hyperactivity in children. However, it has been found that the doses usually prescribed are probably too low to have a noticeable and lasting effect.

Note: Used externally, the oil is helpful for eczema, dry, scaly skin and dandruff, and accelerates wound healing.

For more information about evening primrose oil and its many properties and uses, see Appendix 1, page 327.

GRAPESEED OIL *(Vitis vinifera)*

Like corn oil, grapeseed oil is produced by hot extraction as the seeds are only about 12 per cent oil. The oil can be 'rescued' after steam extraction (before passing through the refining process) but the extra labour and time involved increases the price substantially.

Properties and effects: Grapeseed oil contains a high percentage of linoleic acid and some vitamin E and is one of the few oils that are cholesterol-free and easily digested. It is a gentle emollient, leaving the skin with a satin finish without feeling greasy, therefore preferred for use on oily skin.

HAZELNUT OIL *(Corylus avellana)*

Both male and female flowers are present on each hazel tree. The nut yields an amber yellow oil with a pleasant aroma and a slight flavour of marzipan.
Properties and effects: Oleic acid (a monounsaturated fatty acid) is the principal constituent, with a small proportion of linoliec acid (polyunsaturated fatty acid) also being present.

Hazelnut oil is said to penetrate the top layer of the skin slightly, being beneficial for oily or combination skins and effective on acne. It stimulates the circulation and also has astringent properties. It may be more economical to use it in conjunction with a less expensive base oil. However, when using it to benefit skin disorders, it should be used alone as the base, with added essential oils.

JOJOBA OIL *(Simmondsia chinensis)*

Jojoba (pronounced 'hohoba') is not an oil, but a liquid wax. Jojoba, a desert shrub, is the only plant in the world to contain liquid wax. This replaced sperm whale oil in the cosmetics industry when the whale became an endangered species. It is an environmental aid, as planting it saves arid land from becoming desert – plantations cover over 16,000 hectares in the United States. It is also used instead of beeswax as an emulsifier in creams. Jojoba is very stable, having extremely good keeping qualities as it doesn't contain glycerides and very little fatty acids but does contain 97 per cent wax esters.
Properties and effects: The chemical structure of jojoba not only resembles sebum, but the latter can dissolve in it, which makes it a useful oil for oily skin, especially in cases of acne. Jojoba inhibits the production of excess sebum by imparting a light coating of wax to the skin, thus fooling the body

into believing that enough sebum has been produced. It is this effect that makes jojoba a natural choice for treating acne and dandruff. A balancing oil, it is also indicated for dry scalp and skin, psoriasis and eczema. Jojoba contains an acid (myristic acid) that has anti-inflammatory properties, helpful when mixing a blend for rheumatism and arthritis. In haircare also no other oil can match the ability of jajoba oil to make hair look and feel healthy, as it forms a thin coating on the hair, giving it strength and lustre.

MELISSA OIL – MACERATED *(Melissa officinalis)*

Macerated melissa oil is only produced in regions where melissa is grown for distillation and tea production.

Properties and effects: Melissa oil is indicated for massage on 'heavy legs' (fluid retention), especially in combination with cypress essential oil. It is also beneficial on dry mature skins.

OLIVE OIL *(Olea europaea)*

Traditionally used for centuries in cooking and healing, virgin pressed olive oil is popular on supermarket shelves because of its monounsaturated fatty acid content, effective in the prevention of high cholesterol and heart disease, as well as its wonderful flavour. Its green colour is due to the small percentage of chlorophyll in the flesh of the olive, from which the oil is taken. It is an ideal cooking oil for health-conscious people.

Properties and effects: Externally olive oil is emollient, soothing to inflamed skin and good for sprains and bruises. It is a little heavy for massage, but can be added 50:50 to a less viscous oil.

When ingested, it is not only prophylactic against heart disease, but is a help against hyperacidity and constipation.

PEACH KERNEL OIL *(Prunus persica)*

See: Apricot kernel oil

PEANUT OIL *(Arachis hypogeae)*

Peanut oil has less stable keeping qualities and has quite a noticeable aroma (not unpleasant and not as strong as coconut). It is mostly available only in the refined state although a small quantity is cold-pressed in France.

Properties and effects: A hypoallergenic and emollient oil (particularly for arthritis and sunburn), peanut, while too oily to use on its own for massage, is perfectly acceptable for self-application to specific areas or to blend with another less viscous carrier oil.

ROSEHIP OIL *(Rosa canina; R. mollis)*

Coming mostly from wild plants, this oil is usually organic and yields a lovely golden-red oil, often obtained, unfortunately, by solvent extraction.

Properties and effects: Research in Chile shows rosehip oil to be a tissue regenerator (perhaps due to its high unsaturated fatty acid content), making it an excellent oil for a mature skin. It has been shown to be effective on scars, wounds, burns (including sunburn), eczema and ageing.

SAFFLOWER OIL *(Carthamus tinctorius)*

Safflower, like sunflower, belongs to the Compositae/Asteraceae family and has an orangey-yellow flower. Safflower seeds have been discovered in 3000-year-old Egyptian tombs and both the flowers and seeds have been used in the past as dye.

Properties and effects: Yet another oil high in polyunsaturated fatty acids, safflower helps a number of circulatory problems and, taken internally, is said to be helpful for bronchial asthma. It is beneficial on painful, inflamed joints, sprains and bruises. It is one of the less stable oils (except when it is refined, when it has preservatives added to it).

SESAME OIL *(Sesamum indicum)*

The seeds of the sesame plant are contained inside a long nut and give a high yield of clear pale yellow oil when cold-pressed.

Properties and effects: The pressed oil is rich in vitamins and minerals, its vitamin E and sesamol content giving the oil excellent stability.

It is beneficial for dry skin, psoriasis and eczema and protects the skin to a certain extent from the harmful rays of the sun.

SOYBEAN OIL *(Glycine soja)*

Soybean oil is usually obtained by solvent extraction, as the beans have low oil content. Prone to oxidation, it can be a sensitiser, so it may be wise not to use it in aromatherapy.

SUNFLOWER OIL *(Helianthus annuus)*

Although most sunflower oil is solvent-extracted, we can obtain an oil from organically grown plants that is cold-pressed. This oil has a lovely light texture and is very pleasant to use, leaving the skin with a satin-smooth, non-greasy feel.

Properties and effects: Sunflower oil contains vitamins A, B, D and E (the principal one) and is high in unsaturated fatty acids, making it helpful against arteriosclerosis. It has a prophylactic effect on the skin and is beneficial to leg ulcers, bruises and skin diseases. Sunflower oil has diuretic properties, is expectorant and one of its constituents, inulin, is used in the treatment of asthma.

The leaves and flowers have been used in Russia for years against chest problems such as bronchitis.

WHEATGERM OIL *(Triticum vulgare)*

Wheatgerm oil is of a rich orangey-brown colour and due to its high vitamin E content, widely used to increase the keeping qualities of less stable oils – a minimum of 10 per cent should be added to the base oil, up to 20 per cent if the oil has low stability.

Properties and effects: Wheatgerm is useful on dry and mature skins, though too heavy to use by itself for massage. Taken internally, it is said to help prevent varicose veins, eczema and indigestion, and helps to remove cholesterol deposits from the arteries.

Caution: As it is from a protein, it could be contraindicated for anyone prone to allergies.

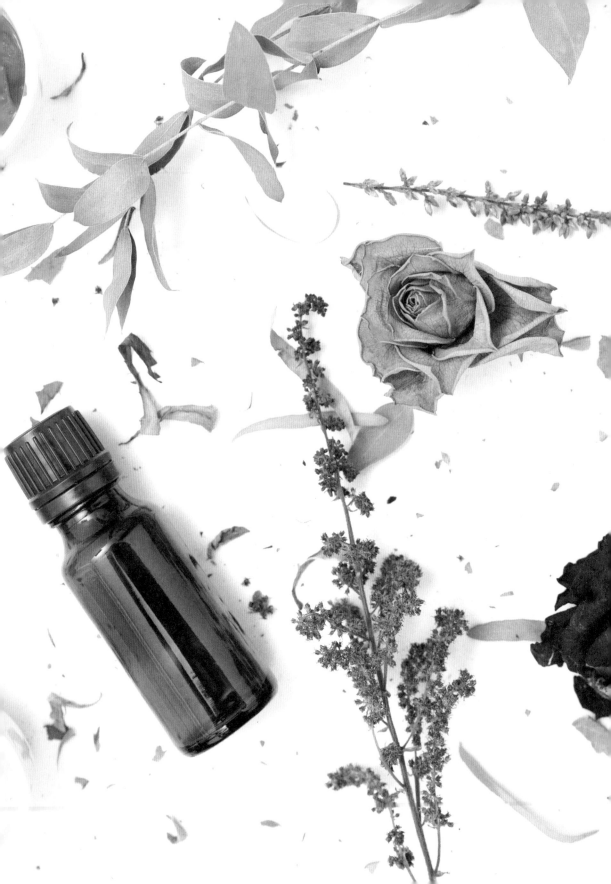

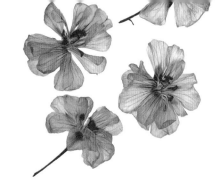

PART II

USING ESSENTIAL OILS IN AROMATHERAPY

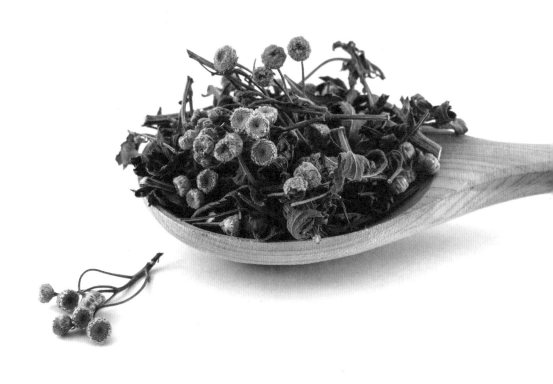

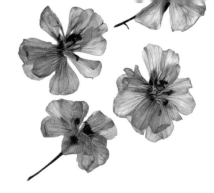

BLENDING
AROMATHERAPY OILS

Pure essential oils are powerful, concentrated substances. They are normally used in very small quantities and diluted in a carrier oil or lotion prior to use on the skin. This facilitates easy application, absorption and ensures against a skin reaction. For an aromatherapy formulations, we choose essential oils and carrier oils as per our specific requirements, depending on our assessment of the client.

BLENDING

The art of blending aromatherapy oils depends on your ability to mix different complementary aromas to heal mind, body and spirit.

Essential oils are synergists, complementing and enhancing each other's therapeutic actions. For this reason, blends of 3 to 5 essential oils are usually recommended for optimum therapeutic effect. To create your own blend, choose oils to suit your client's emotional and physical needs, favouring those with an aroma that appeals to everybody. Mix well and label clearly. Do not attempt to include more than 5 oils in a blend, since this may detract from their synergistic qualities.

Selecting the right essential oil

The most important part of any therapy is 'diagnosis': assessing
the cause of the problem then choosing the right medicine
for the problem. Aromatherapy is no different. Essential oils
are highly versatile in their therapeutic effect, meaning that
a single oil may work for multiple conditions. For the ease of
choosing right oils for blending, we first assess the conditions
that need to be addressed, then classify these conditions
according to importance into:

Primary   Secondary   Tertiary

Now list all the essential oil options available to you for each
condition. Prepare a table format and from this table prefer the
specialist oil suitable for each condition needing maximum
attention. Prefer oils that are common for more than one
condition. Thus choosing between three to five essential oils
for your blend. This way you cannot go wrong in your blends.
However always remember any cautions applying to any oil.

You can also choose your base or carrier oils the same way.

RATIO OR DOSAGE

Essential oils are used in small quantities – almost 2% in a blend. Since
it is difficult to measure very small quantities by weight/volume, they are
measured in terms of the number of drops. Depending upon the viscosity
of the oil, 1 millilitre may contain 20–30 drops. So the easy way of
calculating how much essential oil to add to a base oil is to measure the
amount of base oil in millilitres and then add about half that number of
drops of essential oil.

For example:

- To a 50 ml bottle of base oil, add about 25 drops of essential oil – this gives approximately 2–2.5% dilution. Add a few more drops for a physical remedy, a few less for the treatment of sensitive or facial skin or an emotional or psychological problem.
- To 1 tablespoon (approximately 15 ml) base oil add 6–9 drops of essential oil.
- To 1 teaspoon (approximately 5 ml) carrier oil add 2–3 drops of essential oil.

OIL-BLENDING EQUIPMENT

As well as the essential oils (equipped with dropper plugs) and a range of base oils, you require the following to start blending.

Measuring cylinder: Measuring cylinders, cups and jars are available in various sizes from suppliers of laboratory equipment. If you are doing small quantities, go for the small size cylinders such as 100 millilitres with calibrations for each millilitre. For bigger batches you can go up to 500 millilitres, which may have calibrations for every 10 millilitres.

Stirring rod: Glass stirring rods are required to stir the blends.

Storage bottles: Store the blended oils in dark-coloured glass bottles, preferably with dropper plugs and caps.

Labels: All blends should be correctly labelled, try to incorporate a reference number and date of preparation.

Cleansing alcohol: An alcohol like isopropyl alcohol (sold as rubbing alcohol in pharmacies) is useful for cleaning your equipment.

Cleansing towels: All bottles, equipment and the table should be wiped after making your blends. The stickiness may spoil labels, attract dirt and make the place slippery and messy.

BASIC RULES OF BLENDING

There are certain basic rules to blending an aromatherapy formulation:

- Work out your quantities before you begin.
- List all the essential and carrier oils required with dosages.
- Take out all the essential and base oils and place on the blending table.
- Check all oils for any cautions, as well as rancidity or oxidation. If you feel that there is a change in the smell of the oil or if the oil is looking turbid, do not use it.
- Ensure that your measuring container is clean: the best way to clean the measuring glass or cylinders is with ethyl alcohol or isopropyl alcohol. Because all essential oils dissolve easily in alcoholic solutions, even the residual base will dissolve. You can recycle this solvent at least a few times before throwing it out or using it in a solution as a room scent/freshener.
- Keep the clean bottles ready for filling with the blended oil. Label immediately after filling.
- Close all caps and plugs tightly.
- Wipe all the surfaces immediately and ensure there is no spilled oil residue, as the surface will get stained.
- Do not use or handle any plastic material, as neat essential oils react with plastics.

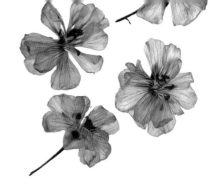

AROMATHERAPY APPLICATIONS AND METHODS OF USE

BATH

This is the easiest and most popular way of using essential oils. A few drops of a natural essential oil mix added to bathwater improves the body's immune level at a physical level, and the oil fragrance works at a mental level by inhalation during the bath.

Different essential oils can be selected for their specific effect – for example, a lemongrass/rosemary blend is uplifting and stimulating, lavender/geranium is soothing and relaxing, and juniper berry helps in relieving fluid retention.

Simply add up to 5 drops in a bucket or up to 15 drops in the bathtub of the chosen blend of pure essential oils. In the case of a shower, keep a full mug of water handy and add 5 drops essential oil, pouring it over yourself once you finish the shower.

Essential oils can also be mixed in a teaspoon of vegetable oil (such as sweet almond oil) before adding to the bath. This helps to moisturise the skin and ensures an even distribution of the essential oils, which is important in the case of babies and young children. However, it may cause greasiness in the bathroom, making it slippery. Therefore it's advisable to use a moisturising blend afterwards.

To avoid possible irritation, always check the safety data, before using a new oil in the bath.

Prepare a few blends and keep them ready. Here are two blends that are good to have on hand: the uplifting blend will prepare you for the day ahead, while the relaxing blend is useful to relieve tension and restore harmony at the end of a stressful day.

Uplifting bath oil	Relaxing bath oil
3 ml of lemon	3 ml of lavender
2 ml of basil	2 ml of clary sage
2 ml of juniper berry	2 ml of geranium
1 ml of peppermint	1 ml of patchouli
1 ml of geranium	1 ml of sandalwood

For each recipe, blend the essential oils in a brown-glass dropper bottle. Screw the bottle lids tightly shut, shake well, and label clearly.

MASSAGE

Massage is a therapy in its own right, and using essential oils adds to the benefit. According to Hippocrates it can 'loosen a stiff joint' or 'bind a loose joint'. Therapeutic massage is the main method used by professional aromatherapists and also in various spa treatments for relaxation and detoxification. In aromatherapy massage, the focus of the therapist should be on the movement and drainage of lymph. If it is not possible to carry out a full body massage, then a foot massage using appropriate oils is an excellent alternative. When we massage the feet, we stimulate the rest of the body as well. This is because all the organs, glands and muscles in the human body have nerve endings located in the soles of the feet. That's how the foot reflexology works.

Massage works on us in multiple ways. Not only it is a touch therapy that helps to soothe the mind and emotions, massage also improves blood circulation, resulting in:

- More nutrients reaching skin surface and helping rejuvenation of the skin.
- Helping to eliminate toxins at the fundamental level, therefore helping to detoxify the body.
- Helping to tone the muscles.

Prime factors for massage

Body massage is a well-orchestrated movement of hands. Different parts of the world practise different kind of massage movement and techniques, however the popular types include Swedish massage, shiatsu, Indian Ayurvedic massage and Thai massage. Whatever type of massage you practise, there are certain prime factors which should be taken into consideration.

Contact: When two energies come into contact initially there is a feeling of shock, then they harmonise. Therefore the contact, once established, should not be broken unless and until it's necessary, for example, to shift the posture. In the process of massage, every time the contact is interrupted and re-established, there is a disturbance of energy that interferes in the relaxation of the client, which is the ultimate objective of the massage.

Continuity: Once started, the massage process should not be interrupted for anything. Therefore all pending work should be taken care of, and ensure you and the client have visited the toilet. Switching off mobile (cell) phones is also recommended.

Pressure: Pressure is an integral part of a massage. But each body type can tolerate a different amount of pressure: some bodies are very delicate; while they may not look that way, they can take only a little pressure, while someone with a delicate-looking body may ask for more pressure. Therefore it is important to ascertain the amount of pressure your client can take. In a severe pain condition use just gentle rubbing or moderate pressure, even if your client asks for more.

Rhythm: Rhythm comes out of experience. Rhythmic massage, like rhythmic music, is soothing and energising.

Speed: The speed of your hand movement determines whether your massage is relaxing or energising. Slow, gentle movements help to relax the mind and body while fast movements are good to energise the body as they improve circulation.

Basic massage movements

Aromatherapy massages do not require any of the 'hacking' or 'cupping' movements required for Swedish massage. It works with gentle movements, however, all movements are directed towards the heart or to the nearest lymph nodes. Basic massage movements include the following steps:

1. **Effleurage:** A stroking movement performed with palms pushing the tissues with pressure towards the heart. Hands should be relaxed and in contact with the soft tissues using firm but gentle pressure. Once contact is made it must be maintained, keeping motion continuous and placing one hand on the body before removing the other, thus ending each sequence. Effleurage improves circulation, helps to spread the essential oils and enables the client to get accustomed to the masseur.

2. **Petrissage:** forms the main and longest part of massage in aromatherapy. It includes the following movements:

    Kneading: this is a circular movement done with the surface of the palms or the thumbs; the pressure is determined depending on the area. This movement helps to break down muscle tension as well as fatty deposits.

Picking up: Here the tissue is 'picked-up' from the bones: the muscles are lifted, squeezed and relaxed without losing contact with the body. The tissues are lifted and moved alternatively, backward and forward in a smooth rolling movement, parallel to the bones. This movement is especially beneficial to reduce fatty tissues.

Wringing: This is similar to picking up but a much stronger movement, like wringing a towel. The flesh is lifted and wrung between both the hands. This is performed mostly on large muscle, for example thighs, calves and buttocks.

3. **Friction**: This helps to break down 'knotted' muscles. It also soothes nerve endings as well as aiding the distribution of fluid around joints, for example, the ankles. The movement involves the thumb working in circles with pressure in an upward motion only.

   Note: friction is combined with or followed by lymphatic drainage. Friction helps in moving the flow of lymph and blood, which should be drained to the nearest lymphatic nodes.

Manual lymphatic drainage (MLD)

MLD is an advanced therapy in which the practitioner uses a range of specialised and gentle rhythmic pumping techniques to move the fluids under the skin in the direction of the lymph flow. This stimulates the lymphatic vessels, which carry substances vital to the defence of the body and removes waste products. The first visit will include a consultation during which the therapist will recommend the number and frequency of future sessions. Each session will last approximately 1 hour. Where appropriate, the therapist will work in conjunction with the client's medical practitioner.

The benefits of MLD

MLD is both preventative and remedial and can enhance wellbeing. Furthermore, MLD:

- is deeply relaxing
- promotes the healing of fractures, torn ligaments and sprains, and lessens pain
- can improve many chronic conditions such as sinusitus, rheumatoid arthritis, scleroderma, acne and other skin conditions
- may strengthen the immune system
- relieves fluid congestion: swollen ankles, tired puffy eyes and swollen legs due to pregnancy
- is an effective component of the treatment and control of lymphoedema and assists in conditions arising from venous insufficiency
- promotes healing of wounds and burns and improves the appearance of old scars
- minimises or reduces stretch marks.

Other kinds of massage

Aromatic oils can also be rubbed into particular areas of the body to help combat specific complaints: tense, aching shoulders should be kneaded using a soothing massage oil to relax the muscles; stomach-ache or period pain can be eased with a gentle antispasmodic oil applied to the abdomen in a clockwise direction.

Massage can also be a very intimate and sensual experience: between lovers it can bring a new depth to a relationship, as well as enhance sexual enjoyment. Some essential oils, including jasmine, ylang ylang, neroli and rose, are renowned for their aphrodisiac effect.

For the purpose of massage, essential oils are mixed with a base oil or vegetable oil, such as sweet almond, olive or grapeseed oil, before being applied to the body. The dilution should be in the region of 1–3 per cent depending upon the type of oil used and the specific purpose. In general, complaints of a physical nature, such as aching muscles or rheumatism, require a stronger concentration than disorders related to the emotions, like depression or insomnia.

The following blends will nourish the body and mind. The stimulating blend can help to improve poor circulation and will revive someone who is tired or rundown. Keep the soothing blend for evening use, since it will relax and prepare for sleep.

Soothing blend	Stimulating blend
2 drops of geranium	3 drops of lemon
3 drops of lavender	2 drops of rosemary
2 drops of sandalwood	2 drops of juniper berry
1 tablespoon (15 ml) of suitable carrier oil	1 tablespoon (15 ml) of suitable carrier oil

Choose whichever blend appeals to you. Mix the essential oils with the carrier oil and store in a clearly labelled screw-top bottle.

VAPORISATION

Aromatherapy vaporisers are a quick and easy way to make your environment smell beautiful. In a vaporiser, oils are heated gently to evaporate from liquid to gaseous state, filling the room with wonderful aromas. (If you have pets, check with your vet before using vaporised essential oils around them, as some are harmful to them.)

Vaporised oils can be used for a variety of reasons, such as creating a relaxed atmosphere in the home or to uplift and stimulate minds in an office, or to disinfect a sickroom. A penetrating oil like sweet basil, for example, can scent a room and dispel unwanted odours while an antiseptic oil such as eucalyptus can rid a room of germs and, combined with peppermint, will help with respiratory complaints. Insect-repellent aromas like citronella and lemongrass can be used to repel mosquitoes and other insects.

There are many ways to vaporise the oils. You can use an oil burner or an electric diffuser or simply add a few drops of oil to a bowl of hot water placed on a radiator. Avoid applying essential oils directly to a light bulb, as this may cause the bulb to explode. If you wish to keep insects at bay, applying oils to hanging ribbons or to fabric, for example curtains, can be very effective. A few drops of an expectorant and decongestant essential oil such as eucalyptus or myrtle put on the pillow at night will combat coughs and colds. Similarly, a combination of mandarin and marjoram on a pillow will prevent snoring and a combination of clary sage with marjoram will promote peaceful sleep.

SOME USEFUL OILS FOR VAPORISATION

Relaxing	Uplifting	Sedative	Sensual
lavender	lemon	clary sage	jasmine
sandalwood	basil	marjoram	ylang ylang
vetiver	neroli	lavender	patchouli
geranium	rosemary	valerian	cedarwood
mandarin	lemongrass	patchouli	clove

Steam inhalation

An easy way to reap the benefits of essential oils is to inhale them through steam vapours. The faster the oils evaporate, the faster they are breathed in and the faster decongestion occurs. The facial skin also gets cleansed through this process. Steam inhalation involves three simple steps:

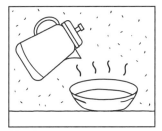 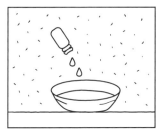 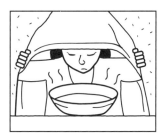

1. Fill a bowl with steaming hot water *2. Add 5–10 drops of chosen essential oils.* *3. Inhale the steam using a towel to seal in the vapours.*

This method is especially suited to decongesting the sinuses, throat and chest. Add 5–10 drops of an essential oil, such as eucalyptus, rosemary or peppermint, or a combination of all three, to a bowl of steaming water, cover the head with a towel and breathe deeply for 3–10 minutes, keeping the eyes closed.

Steam inhalation also acts as a kind of facial 'sauna'. The use of oils such as tea-tree, juniper berry, geranium and lavender can help unblock the pores and clear the complexion of spots and blackheads.

Soaking in a steaming hot bath containing expectorant oils, which are non-irritating to the skin, such as pine needle or marjoram, can also help clear congestion.

Note: Steam inhalations are not recommended for asthma sufferers.

COMPRESS

Compresses are a simple and useful way of treating a wide range of body conditions with aromatherapy essential oils. From cuts, bruises and grazes to sprains, strains, inflammation, fever and more, essential oils used in compresses can help in wide range of problems and aid the recovery process.

Compresses are simply a cloth or hand towel soaked in hot or ice-cold water, to which essential oils are added. Hot and cold compresses are used to treat different conditions and it's important to know when to use which type of compress.

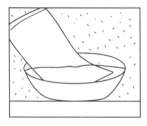 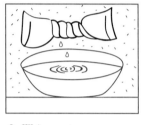 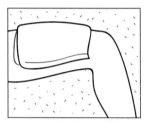

1. Soak a cloth.   *2. Wring out.*   *3. Apply to affected area.*

Hot compresses

Hot compresses increase circulation to the affected area and help to relieve muscular aches and pains, arthritis and rheumatic pain, lower back pain, menstrual pain, frozen shoulder, muscle cramps, cystitis, abscesses etc. You can crush a piece of ginger while heating the water to increase heat and circulation.

Useful oils for hot compresses include eucalyptus, ginger, black pepper, clove, chamomile, lavender, wintergreen and myrtle.

Cold compresses

Cold compresses, especially those incorporating ice, help reduce swelling, can be applied to relieve conditions including bumps, bruises, inflammation, boils, headaches and fever. Useful oils for cold compress include lavender, rosemary, eucalyptus, peppermint and basil.

You can also alternate between hot and cold compresses for conditions including sprains, arthritis and boils.

SITZ BATH

Sitz baths are very useful for urinary, genital and anal complaints including cystitis, pruritus, thrush, haemorrhoids, piles and fistula.

Cystitis, which is an infection of the bladder, is characterised by a painful burning sensation while passing urine. Pruritus, or itching, is an irritating condition that often accompanies a mild vaginal infection. The best help for the condition is a sitz bath with bactericidal oils, two to three times daily. They are easy to make: simply add chosen essential oils to a tub of warm water, in which you can sit. Alternatively you can use a bathtub for the same purpose.

To help combat cystitis and pruritus, add 5–10 drops of any one of the following oils: lavender, juniper, sandalwood, tea-tree, cypress or bergamot, to sitz bathwater, or add 2–3 drops to a bidet for localised washing.

DOUCHE

A douche is a vaginal enema into which we add essential oils. This method can be very helpful in the treatment of vaginal conditions such as leucorrhea or candida (thrush), or any other vaginal infection.

Using a plastic douche or enema pot, add 3–5 drops of any 3 of the following essential oils: tea-tree, sandalwood, palmarosa, cypress, lavender, juniper and geranium, to 500 ml warm water and stir well before inserting.

GARGLE

For the treatment of mouth ulcers, sore throats, bad breath or other mouth or gum infections, simply add about 3 drops of an essential oil such as tea-tree, cypress, clove, bergamot or fennel to a glass of warm boiled water, mix well and gargle.

NEAT APPLICATION

Pure essential oils are strong chemicals and should not be applied neat to the skin. Some oils can cause irritation or a burning or tingling sensation when they are applied in an undiluted form, however, there are exceptions to this rule. Lavender, for example, can be applied directly to burns, insect bites, cuts, cramps and tired or pulled muscles. Tea-tree oil can be used directly on warts and nail bed infections. And in the case of an emergency, like a cut or wound, any oil can be used neat as an antiseptic. Some oils can be used as perfumes (like sandalwood, jasmine, rose and agarwood oil). Otherwise, most oils should not be applied undiluted, unless specifically directed.

PERFUMES

In India and other parts of the worlds attars, or traditional perfumes, are made with natural essential oils. Many essential oils are ideal as perfumes, either on their own or combined with others, such as rose, jasmine, neroli and sandalwood – all very popular scents. Ylang ylang, patchouli, vetiver and geranium are renowned as well-balanced fragrances. They can be dabbed on the wrist or behind the ears (on the pulse points), either neat or diluted in 5% of jojoba (for example 10 drops to 1 teaspoon of oil). Before using a new oil as a perfume, always do a patch test. Aromatic oils can also be used to scent hair, linen, clothes, paper and potpourri – and more.

Pure essential oils have a totally different quality from synthetic perfumes because they are derived from natural sources. Artificially made perfumes do not have the subtle balance of constituents and the therapeutic qualities of real essential oils, and may also cause an allergic reaction in sensitive people.

SKINCARE

Aromatherapy essential oils are ideally suited for skincare, since they are readily absorbed and have the ability to penetrate through to the underlying layers of the skin.

Essential oils stimulate cellular regeneration, improve circulation and help to eliminate toxins at the fundamental level. Therefore skin that has been treated with aromatic oils becomes healthier and more dynamic. Skin and beauty care are central to the practise of aromatherapy – whether by beauty therapists or by laypeople. Most of the aromatic recipes are simple and easy to make at home.

Facial oils

These are blended in the same way as massage oils, except that the carrier oil as well as the essential oil can be adapted to the type of skin being treated. Additional specialised base oils like avocado, jojoba, wheatgerm, hazelnut, rosehip seed, borage seed, macerated carrot and evening primrose may be used, in combination with the basic carrier oils such as sweet almond, grapeseed, sunflower, sesame seed and soybean oil.

An easy recipe is 2 teaspoons (10 ml) of basic carrier oil with 1 teaspoon (5 ml) of specialised carrier oil suited to skin type and 6–8 drops of essential oil. (See also The Face, page 221.)

Facial creams

An aromatic facial cream can be made by adding 8–10 drops of essential oil (according to skin type) to an unscented cream (100 g jar) or by making up a basic cream:

10 g of beeswax

40 g of almond oil

40 g of rosewater or distilled water

10 drops of chosen essential oil

Shred the beeswax and put it into a pyrex (heatproof glass) bowl together with the almond oil. Place the bowl in a double boiler or a pan of water over gentle heat, and mix until the beeswax has melted. Warm the water in the same fashion, and add to the wax and the oil mixture gradually, beating all the time. When the cream mix cools, add the essential oil and stir in, then put in the fridge to set.

This cream can be used for the face, the hands or for massaging the body.

Gels

Natural gels like aloe vera or witch-hazel provide a useful non-oily medium for the application of essential oils as an alternative to oils and creams. A gel can be used to dilute any essential oil for irritating skin conditions, such as eczema or athlete's foot, particularly if the skin is broken, since they prevent the skin forming a crust. This method is also suitable for general skincare, especially if the skin tends to be greasy. Add 2–3 drops of essential oil to a teaspoonful of gel and mix well before applying to the skin.

Masks

Face masks have many benefits – they can nourish, rejuvenate, stimulate, cleanse the skin, and generally improve its texture and quality. Masks can be made from a wide range of natural ingredients including fruit pulp, yoghurt, honey and clay. There are many different types of clay, but green clay, or fuller's earth, is the most versatile, as it is a good antiseptic and rich in minerals. A good basic recipe is 50 g of green clay and 2 teaspoons of cornflour, mixed together and kept in a jar. When you want to make a mask, mix 1 tablespoon of the mask mix with a little water and 3 drops of an essential oil suited to your skin type. Avoid clay masks for dry skin or after aromatherapy treatments unless you add a little base oil to it as it will draw the moisture out of the skin. An essential oil and clay mask is excellent for the treatment of acne and congested skin. Honey is good for revitalising dry complexions and helping to balance combination skin, as well as being generally rejuvenating.

Here are effective and easy recipes for normal to oily skin and for dry skin. Apply the mask once a week to achieve a noticeable improvement in skin texture.

Normal to oily skin	Dry skin
2 drops of juniper	1 drop of sandalwood
1 drop of geranium	1 drop of lavender
1 drop of lavender	1 drop of roman chamomile
2 tsp of live, natural yoghurt	2 tsp of honey

Blend the oils with the yoghurt or honey and spread the mixture lightly and evenly over the face. After a few minutes, when the mask no longer feels cool, rinse off and apply a moisturiser.

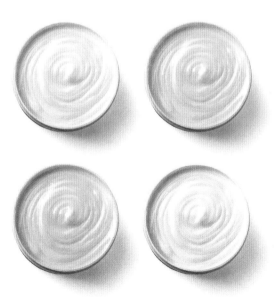

Flower waters

These are easy to make and are beneficial for all types of skin. Simply add up to 100 drops of essential oil to a 500 ml bottle of distilled or rosewater, leave it to stand for up to a month, and then filter using coffee filter paper. Lavender, lemon, rose and neroli are traditional oils used to make floral water but other oils such as geranium or sandalwood may also be used, either individually or blended together.

A variety of essential oils can also be diluted in alcohol to make toilet waters, eau de colognes or aftershave lotions. For example, a traditional toilet water called eau de Portugal can be made by mixing 20 drops of sweet orange, 5 drops of geranium in 1 tablespoon of vodka and 100 ml of spring water. Shake well and leave it to mature for a month, at least, then filter.

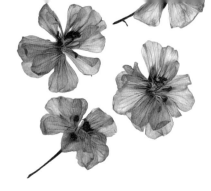

SAFETY GUIDELINES

In general, essential oils are safe to use if used correctly. Experiencing and exploring the unique scents and individual properties of essential oils is both helpful and inspiring. However, because of the high concentration and potency of the oils, it is necessary to take some precautions, as you would with anything unfamiliar.

SAFETY DATA

Always check the specific safety data and caution before using a new oil.

INTERNAL USE

Do not take essential oils internally. This rule is in accordance with the safety guidelines recommended by the International Federation of Aromatherapists. Essential oils don't mix with water, and in an undiluted form they may damage the delicate lining of the digestive tract. In addition, some essential oils are toxic if taken internally. There is a misconception that things taken internally will work faster and better but that is not true: our digestive system is selective and does not absorb everything taken internally, while the skin is a semi-permeable and absorbs up to 40 per cent of essential oils when diluted in light base oils and rubbed on the skin.

NEAT APPLICATION

In general, essential oils should not be applied neat to the skin. They need to be diluted in a carrier oil, gel or cream first. There are exceptions to this rule, such as the use of neat lavender for cuts, spots and burns. Another exception is for emergency use. Certain non-irritant essential oils can also be used as perfumes. Always do a patch test first and keep well away from the eyes.

SKIN IRRITATION

Oils that may irritate the skin or cause an allergic reaction are sweet basil, black pepper, cinnamon, clove bud, eucalyptus, ginger, lemon, lemongrass, peppermint, pine needle and thyme. These oils should be used at half the usual recommended dilutions and no more than 3 drops added to the bath. If irritation does occur, bathe the area with cold water.

SENSITIVE SKIN

Although tea tree oil is sometimes used neat, some oils including tea-tree may cause skin irritation in people with very sensitive skins, so it is important for those with sensitive skins to dilute this useful oil first in a non-oily cream or gel.

PATCH TEST

Always do a patch test before using a new oil check for individual sensitisation. Simply put a few drops on the back of your wrist, cover with a plaster and leave for an hour or more. If irritation or redness occurs, bathe the area with cold water. For further use, reduce the concentration level by half or avoid the oil altogether.

TOXICITY

Essential oils should be used in moderation and externally. Because of high toxicity levels, certain oils like aniseed, camphor, clove bud, hyssop, nutmeg, oregano, sweet fennel and Spanish sage should be avoided or used only in very small dosages.

Hazardous oils such as pennyroyal, mustard, sassafras, rue and mugwort should not be used at all.

PHOTOSENSITIVITY AND TOXICITY

Some oils are phototoxic, which means they cause skin pigmentation if exposed to direct sunlight. Do not use the following oils on the skin, either neat or in dilution, if the area will be exposed to the sun or ultraviolet light (as on a sun bed): bergamot (except bergapten-free oil), angelica, cumin, lemon, lime, mandarin or orange.

BABIES AND CHILDREN

Always dilute oils for babies and infants to at least half the recommended amount. For young children, avoid altogether the possible toxic and irritant oils listed above.

0–12 months: Use only 1 drop of 'safe' oils (non-toxic and non-irritant): lavender, geranium, rose, roman chamomile, neroli or sandalwood diluted in 1 teaspoon of carrier oil for massage or bathing.

1–5 years: Use only 2–3 drops of the aforesaid 'safe' oils diluted in 1 teaspoon carrier oil for massage or bathing.

6–12 years: Use as for adults but in half the stated concentration.

Teenagers: Use as directed for adults.

PREGNANCY

During pregnancy, use essential oils in half the usual stated amount because of the sensitivity of the growing foetus. Oils which are potentially toxic or have hormonal or emmenagogic properties (that is, they stimulate the uterus muscles) are contraindicated.

The following oils should be avoided altogether: Basil, cinnamon leaf, citronella, clary sage, clove, hyssop, juniper, marjoram, myrrh, Spanish sage, tarragon and thyme.

The following oils are best avoided during the first 4 months of pregnancy: Angelica root, Atlas cedarwood, sweet fennel, juniper berry, peppermint and rosemary.

HIGH BLOOD PRESSURE

Avoid the following oils, in cases of this condition, as they can raise the blood pressure: black pepper, cypress, hyssop, rosemary, sage (all types) and thyme.

EPILEPSY

Most of the oils with high ketone and phenol content have a strong aroma that can have a strong effect on the nervous system and may be neurotoxic for epileptics. The following oils should be used with care on epileptics due to their powerful effect on the nervous system: sweet fennel, hyssop, oregano, peppermint, thyme, jasmine and sage.

ALCOHOL

Clary sage and marjoram essential oils should not be used in any form within a few hours of drinking alcohol. This can cause nausea, exaggerated drunkenness and even hallucinations.

HOMEOPATHY

Homeopathic treatment is not compatible with the following oils due to their strength: black pepper, camphor, eucalyptus and peppermint.

STORAGE

Store in dark bottles, away from light and heat, and well out of reach of children.

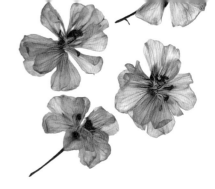

USING AROMATHERAPY WITH OTHER THERAPIES

All holistic therapies have been dubbed 'alternative therapies'. In fact they are all complementary therapies and two or three systems of healing can be combined. The job of the healer is not to prove the supremacy of one therapy over another, but to heal the client. The use of essential oils is part of some of the ancient therapies, such as Ayurveda, however, essential oils can also be combined even with modern medicine in many ways. Also, naturopathy, acupressure, reiki, pranic healing and other energy-healing techniques can make use of the healing properties and high vibrations of the natural essential oils. I use essential oils for the healing of chakras and have created chakra anointments.

CHAKRA HEALING WITH ESSENTIAL OILS

What human beings are to the animal world, a tree is to the plant kingdom. The five elements and three guna that we associate with various chakras are also represented in plants. For that reason, Ayurveda classifies certain plants and oils more Sattvic (purer, with high vibrations) than others.

The five basic elements in plants and the use of their essences for chakra healing are:

Earth: As the earth element is associated with our root chakra, in plants it is associated with the roots. Similarly, the oils from various plant roots are used to energise and balance the base root, or muladhar, chakra. Jatamansi (Indian spikenard) is a renowned essential oil used for muladhar as well as crown chakra imbalances. Other useful oils include angelica root, valerian root, costus root, nagarmotha (*Cyperus scariosus*), patchouli and vetiver.

Water: Although associated with swadhisthan, or the sacral chakra, the water element is associated with the trunk of the plant, since trunks work as waterways for the entire plant. Most useful among the oils for the sacral chakra are sandalwood, cedarwood, rose wood and ginger (a modified stem).

Fire: The fire element is represented in our solar plexus, or manipura chakra. It is associated with brightly coloured flowers and spices such as black pepper and clove. Other useful oils include rosemary, marjoram, chamomiles, lavender, thyme, fennel, cardamom, rose, geranium and clary sage.

Air: The air element present in our heart (anahat) chakra is represented in plants through their leaves. The most revered plant for the heart chakra is holy basil. Other useful plant oils include eucalyptus, peppermint, lotus, rose, tea-tree, lemongrass, rosemary, frankincense, lavender and thyme.

Ether: Described as 'space' or 'akash tattva' (element), ether is associated with our vishuddha or throat chakra. In plants, this element is associated with the fruits and the seeds. The useful oils are lemon, orange, bergamot, bayberry, sandalwood, lotus, tea-tree etc.

As our third eye chakra represents all the five basic elements (panch mahabhoot), plant seeds also represent all the five elements. As a seed is a potential plant, the seed oils can be used on all the chakras according to their property.

The essential oils should be diluted in a suitable base oil. Lotus seed or black til (sesame seed) oil is considered as Sattvic base oils, to be used for chakra anointments. You can also combine oils for each chakra according to the therapeutic effect on the associated organs and glands or as per their colour vibrations. The selection and dosage should be as per the assessment of a qualified therapist with an understanding of chakra imbalances. If unsure, use pre-blended anointments from a trusted source.

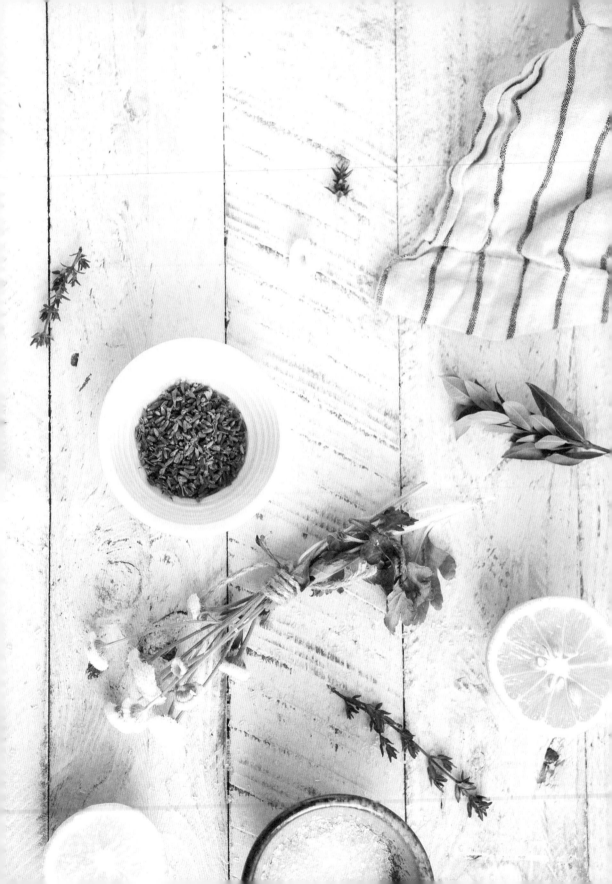

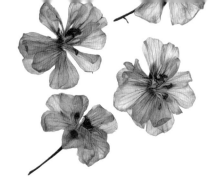

FIFTY EASY WAYS TO USE AROMATHERAPY/ ESSENTIAL OILS

1. Baths are the easiest and most versatile way to use essential oils. They work at the physical as well as psychological level. At the physical level, they boost the immune system while at the psychological level they affect mental/emotional state. Lavender and geranium are the most versatile all-rounders and can be used alone or in combination with other oils.

2. Keep hypertension at bay by using a combination of lavender, geranium and sandalwood oil as a relaxing bath oil (5 drops in a bucket or 12–15 in a bathtub). This will also boost immunity levels.

3. To lift mood and overcome depression, use a combination of lemongrass, bergamot, geranium or neroli and rosemary in the bath (5 drops in a bucket or 12–15 in a bathtub), or vaporise.

4. Add a few drops of essential oils of lemongrass, rosemary or lemon to water in a spray bottle and use as an air freshener. You can also add rosemary, frankincense and holy basil to cleanse the energy around, as these oils repel negative energies.

5. To disinfect your home or a patient's room, use a few drops of

eucalyptus, lemon, cinnamon, pine, geranium and tea-tree, either in a vaporiser or water sprayer.

6. Overindulged last night? Essential oils of juniper, cedarwood, grapefruit, lavender, fennel, rosemary, peppermint and lemon help soften the effects of a hangover. Make your own blend using 3–5 of these oils and use a total of 5–6 drops in a bath.

7. Relieve muscle cramps with neat lavender application. For tired aching muscles or arthritis aches, mix 1 drop each of eucalyptus, wintergreen, lavender, rosemary, sage or basil oil to 1 tablespoon of olive or other vegetable oil and use as a massage oil.

8. Ease headache/migraine pain by rubbing a drop of lavender with a touch of peppermint oil onto your forehead and the back of your neck.

9. To blend your own massage oil: add 3–5 drops of your favourite essential oils such as lavender, geranium or sandalwood to 1 tablespoon of jojoba or other skin-nourishing vegetable oil.

10. As first aid for cuts, burns, bumps, insect bites and even cramps or sprains, use a combination of lavender, tea-tree and German chamomile.

11. For urinary infections, use a combination of tea-tree, sandalwood, palmarosa and juniper berry in a sitz bath.

12. Smelly and sweaty feet can be remedied by either dropping a few drops of pine needle, cypress and geranium essential oils directly into the shoes or by placing a cotton ball dabbed with a few drops of lemon oil into the shoes. Or use the oils in a footbath.

13. For leucorrhoea and candida (thrush), use tea-tree and a lemon oil/bergamot oil combination in a sitz bath or douche.

14. For quick relief from mouth ulcers, dab on 1 drop of tea-tree oil two to three times a day.

15. For bad breath use a combination of bergamot, geranium, tea-tree and spearmint oil mixed with water for a gargle, twice daily.

16. For quick relief from laryngitis and pharyngitis, use a combination of

sandalwood, tea-tree, lemon and bergamot oil: use a few drops mixed with warm water for a gargle two to three times daily.

17. Apply true lavender oil and tea-tree oil directly to cuts, scrapes or scratches. One or two drops will promote healing.

18. Lavender, clary sage and marjoram promote sleep and relieve insomnia: use a few drops on your pillow or the collar/neck of nightclothes.

19. Lavender helps reduce blood pressure and hypertension and can also be good first aid for a heart attack patient – rub on chest and soles of feet.

20. Dab acne/pimples or any boil with tea-tree oil for a quick result.

21. Place 1 drop of peppermint oil in half a glass (125 ml) of water and sip slowly to relieve hot flushes. It also aids digestion and relieves upset stomach.

22. For quick relief from asthma attack, inhale peppermint oil.

23. For any skin allergy, use lavender oil with a few drops of water.

24. Use a combination of lavender, marjoram and clary sage in a vegetable oil massaged on the lower abdomen to relieve menstrual cramps.

25. One drop of tea-tree or oregano essential oil applied directly to a wart is an effective means of elimination. You can also make a mix of tea-tree and oregano in jojoba oil. Apply the essential oil blend daily until the wart is gone.

26. For a nail bed infection, use a drop of tea-tree oil for a few days until it's gone.

27. Rosemary oil helps people suffering from low blood pressure: use in bath or massage.

28. Rosemary and holy basil oils promote alertness and stimulate memory. Inhale occasionally during long car trips and while reading or studying.

29. To relieve anxiety, lie down on a bed and use a few drops of lavender oil on your solar plexus. Parents can use it for their children.

30. For quick relief for sprained and stiff muscles, apply lavender oil directly.

31. Potpourri that has lost its scent can be revived by adding a few drops of essential oil. Add patchouli and sandalwood for a longer-lasting effect.

32. The bathroom is easily scented by placing oil-scented cotton balls in inconspicuous places, or sprinkle oils directly onto silk or dried flower arrangements or wreaths.

33. Essential oils or blends make wonderful perfumes. Create your own personal essence using 25 drops of essential oils to 2 tablespoons of perfume alcohol. Let it age two weeks before using.

34. An essential oil dropped on a radiator, scent ring or lamp will not only fill the room with a wonderful fragrance, but will also set a mood such as calming or uplifting.

35. When moving into a new home, first use a water spray containing a combination of basil, sage, rosemary and frankincense essential oils. They will cleanse the aura and change the odour environment to your own. Do this for several days until it begins to feel like your space.

36. To bring fever down, sponge the body with cool water to which 1 drop each of eucalyptus, peppermint and lavender oils have been added.

37. Jojoba oil makes an ideal hair nourisher for coloured hair, without affecting the colour. It can also be used on eyebrows.

38. When washing out the fridge, freezer or oven, add 1 drop of lemon, lime, grapefruit, bergamot, mandarin, or orange essential oil to the final rinse water.

39. To dispel mosquitoes and other picnic or barbecue pests, drop a few drops of lemongrass or citronella oil with camphor in the melted wax of a candle or place a few drops on the barbecue hot coals.

40. Infuse bookmarks and stationery with essential oils. It will save them from moths and silverfish. Place drops of oil on paper and put them in a plastic bag, seal it and leave overnight to infuse the aroma. Send only good news in perfumed letters.

41. Use 1 drop Roman chamomile oil on a cloth-wrapped ice cube to relieve teething pain in children.

42. To fragrance your kitchen cabinets and drawers, place a 'food scent' or lemon oil dabbed on a cotton ball in an inconspicuous corner. To repel cockroaches, use a camphor and eucalyptus combination.

43. Add 1 drop each of lavender, geranium and sandalwood oil to your facial moisturiser to bring out a radiant glow in your skin.

44. Place 1 or 2 drops of rosemary or ylang ylang on your hairbrush before brushing to promote growth and thickness.

45. To enjoy a scented candle, place a drop or two of essential oil into the hot melted wax as the candle burns.

46. To dispel household cooking odours, add a few drops of clove or cinnamon oil to a simmering pan.

47. A drop of lemon essential oil on a soft cloth will polish copper with gentle buffing.

48. Putting a few drops of your favourite essential oil on a cotton ball and placing it in your vacuum cleaner bag will give a pleasant odour to your room. Lemongrass, eucalyptus, rosemary and geranium are nice.

49. A wonderful massage blend for babies is 1 drop of Roman chamomile, 1 drop of lavender and 1 drop of geranium diluted in 2 tablespoons (30 ml) of sweet almond oil and 1 tablespoon (15 ml) of grapeseed oil.

50. For scent-sational-smelling towels, sheets, clothes etc. place a few drops of lavender, geranium or any other chosen essential oil onto a small piece of terry cloth and toss into the clothes dryer while drying. Add 5 drops essential oil to a quarter of a cup (60 ml) of fabric softener or water and place in the centre cup of the wash.

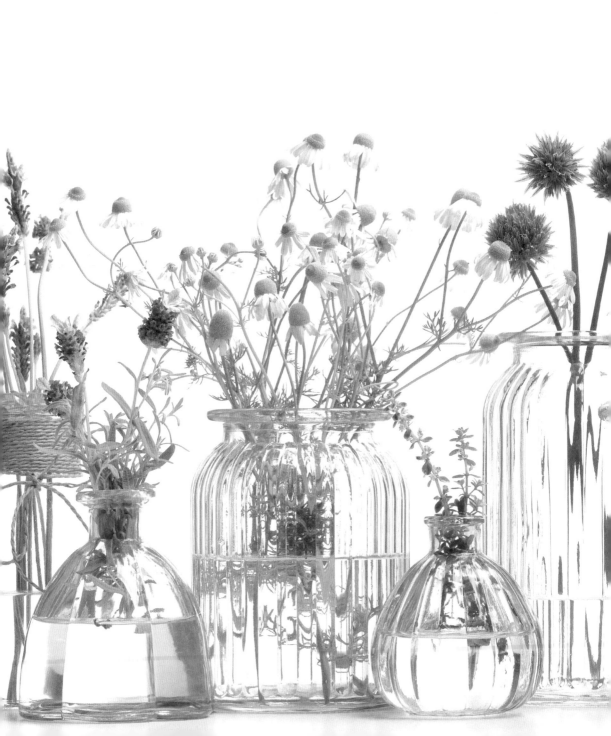

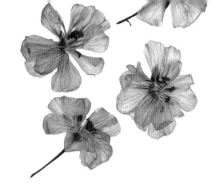

PART III

AROMATIC BODY AND BEAUTY THERAPY

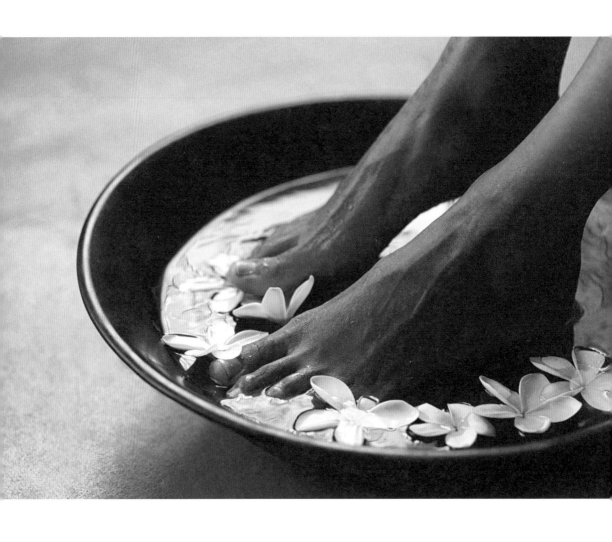

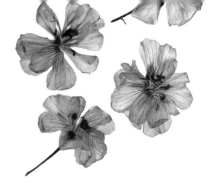

THE CONCEPT OF HEALTH AND BEAUTY

This section is designed to examine various aspects of health and beauty. The balancing, cleansing and regenerative qualities of essential oils bring about a harmony of mind and body as well as a healthy glow to the skin.

According to the ancient law of the 'microcosm and macrocosm' there is no real difference between the vast external universe and the limited universe of the human body. A human being is the living microcosm of the universe and the universe is the macrocosm of a human being. According to kundalini tantra, the human body is composed of three layers (bodies), which function as the vehicle for the inner self. These are not bodies in the physical sense; rather a kind of energy sheath or vibratory field, which embodies the underlying consciousness. The physical body, this body we normally experience and sustain with food, originates in the sexual union of the parents. Our awareness within this body constitutes the waking state of consciousness. It is made up of 16 components: five sensory organs, five organs of action, five elements, and the mind. The energetic basis or pure form of the physical body is the subtle or astral body, represented as our aura. The subtle body is also composed of 16 components. Within the subtle body exist the seven major chakras, known as psychic energy centres. Chakras, the energy centres, are transfer points for our thoughts and emotions, and affect the physical functioning of our endocrine glands and vital organs. Chakra activity is affected by our mental and emotional state, so when they are balanced we feel maximum vitality in health and body (intense happiness). Daily stress can result in chakra imbalances and physical, physiological and emotional disorders.

HOLISTIC HEALTH

Our health is not just the absence of disease, rather it's the balance of the mind, body and spirit. According to Ayurveda, the ancient Indian science of health and healing, it's the balance of five elements: earth, water, fire, air and ether; three gunas: tamas, rajas and sattva; and three doshas: kapha, pitta and vata.

There are two concepts of medicine which are complementary to each other, though head and tail of the same coin. Orthodox medicine (allopath) or classical medicine looks on sickness as 'accidental' – a combination of signals and symptoms due to an exterior damaging agent. However, a complementary therapist would see the symptoms in the light of the whole being – as clues to causes of the disease and treat this rather than symptoms. The cause may lie in any of the different aspects of patient's lifestyle: physical/ physiological, nutritional, mental/emotional or social/ spiritual.

A healthy lifestyle is the guarantee of long-lasting vigor and vitality. By following a healthy regimen you can promote health and avoid disease. The holistic approach is to look for the underlying causes of the disease by analysing a person's lifestyle and to treat these elements rather than symptoms. Over 80 per cent of health problems can be taken care of at home until they become chronic. Therefore it's important to look into the different aspects of the patient's lifestyle:

Emotional lifestyle: Psycho-neuro-immunology, a fairly new discipline, is the study of thoughts and how they can influence the brain and directly affect health of our cells in all parts of the body and one's whole outlook on

As an extension, much emphasis is placed on the relationship between our health and emotional state: 'We are what we think' – happy, positive thoughts exert a positive influence on both health and life in general, whereas negative emotions are self-inflicted wounds, which effectively close down the immune system, leaving the body vulnerable to a wide range of psychosomatic disorders.

Mental attitude plays a far greater part in day-to-day health than is realised. For those who find positive thinking difficult or do not have faith strong enough to believe that things can be changed, essential oils are an alternative route, as essential oils affect our health from the same starting point as our thoughts – the pituitary and the pineal body, the seat of the mind and emotions.

Nutritional lifestyle: The saying 'You are what you eat' is indeed true. Diet and nutrition is an important factor for a healthy life. Incorrect eating habits can be a cause of poor health.

Physical lifestyle: Physical regimen also is a key to good health. Light exercise such as yoga or tai chi have soma psychic (body over mind) effect and ease depression, assist in bowel movement and promote sound sleep. Exercise tones muscles, strengthens bones, makes the heart and lungs work better and increases our physical reserve and vitality. Some people achieve the amount of exercise required from their normal routine while those who lead a sedentary lifestyle are prone to illness.

Social lifestyle: A person's social lifestyle also contributes to their wellbeing. While belonging to a peer group or social circle leads to good health, living in solitude or heavy smoking/drinking regularly in groups or solitude is harmful for health.

Spiritual lifestyle: Spirituality is the science of the self. Our spiritual practices help us to manage our stress much better. You may notice that those who are truly spiritual have a certain radiance about them and they are much more in control of their mind and emotions. An assessment of spiritual lifestyle is an important part of health assessment and guidance.

A complementary therapist has to look into all these aspects of a patient's lifestyle. Every disease can be cured but not every patient. Some people may enjoy being ill so don't really want to be cured, enjoying the sympathy and attention given to them. This is mostly a result of a longstanding imbalance or insecurity.

HOLISTIC BEAUTY

This is the beauty of the whole individual, not just outer beauty that is only skin-deep. Real beauty merges inner beauty (which we can call spirit or love or compassion) with outer beauty, which is our physical body. The most beautiful woman is the one blessed with an attractive physical appearance, but above and beyond this, she radiates love, joy, contentment and good health.

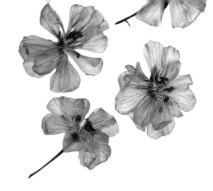

UNDERSTANDING OUR SKIN

One of the greatest treasures that a person can have is healthy radiant skin. Our skin is the mirror of our health. A beautiful complexion and glorious skin are a reflection of our personal lifestyle practices and inner health. In fact, inner health is the sum total of our lifestyles – physical, nutritional, mental/emotional, social and spiritual.

The skin is a living organ and the largest of the body's organs. The whole skin of an adult has an area of about 2 square metres. In total it weighs about 3 kilograms. Just 6.5 square centimetres has 94 sebaceous glands, 60 hairs, 19,000 sensory nerve cells, 1250 pain receptors and about 17 metres of blood vessels.

It is made up of two main layers: the **epidermis,** which is what you can see, and the **dermis.** The epidermis makes up the top half-millimetre or so. Beneath this is the dermis, about 2 millimetres thick. Millions of dividing cells at the base of the epidermis push wave after wave of new cells towards the surface. Closer to the surface, they are squashed flat and this flexible pavement of dead cells is waterproof. The outer layer protects by sealing in all the body's fluids and keeping out anything potentially harmful. The inner layer supports, nourishes and supplies the outer with that most essential commodity – moisture.

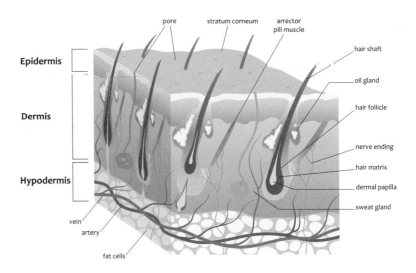

3D section of the skin.

In structure the two layers are different. The epidermis consists of several rows of living cells covered by compact sheets of dead cells (sometimes referred to as the keratin layer). It is constantly growing and about every 20 days new cells are born at its base. They quickly die and dead cells are then pushed to the surface by the arrival of the new ones underneath and are continuously shed. Every new top layer is another chance to have beautiful skin. Even if you remove a portion of the outer layer, it will grow back as good as new. The dermis gives the skin its strength and ability to stretch. It is here that vital nerves, glands, hair follicles and blood vessels are to be found. Skin contains millions of sensitive nerve endings, which tell the brain about touch, temperature, pressure and pain. Sebaceous glands produce oil, called sebum, which keeps the skin supple and waterproof. The different structures in the skin work together to help control the body's temperature and receive touch sensations.

The living reproductive cells are nourished through the blood vessels, but the dead cells have only one requirement: water, which plumps, softens or smooths them. The amount of water the outer layer holds determines the skin's texture and to some extent its contour. It receives a steady supply of water from the dermis, but this is limited and frequently not enough. The epidermis also holds the skin's pigment: the darker the skin, the greater the pigmentation. Oil and sweat glands are situated below but communicate to the outer layer through ducts that end on the surface. Oil glands greatly influence the skin condition and skin type.

Our skin serves the body in many ways, including:

- Sensory perception
- Protecting underlying tissues from injury and dehydration
- Assisting in processes of temperature maintenance and toxic waste elimination
- Serving as the origination point for the manufacture of vitamin D
- Giving structure to all organs and systems within the body.

Ultimately our skin is an integral part of our being and plays a vital role within the body's supportive and functional capacities. It is essential that we learn to take care of it and nourish it so that it will remain healthy regardless of the climate we live in or our chronological age. Truly beautiful skin is always the result of a healthy, stress-free lifestyle and regular nourishing and cleansing. Nature has blessed us with a variety of products including essential and base oils used in aromatherapy and other wholesome ingredients, many of which are available in our kitchen cupboard or fridge or available easily from a natural products supplier. You can use these ingredients to create a variety of products to both cleanse and nourish your skin, hair, nails and more.

SKIN TYPES

There are three skin types: oily, dry and balanced (normal). Many skins are a combination of oily and dry. What your skin needs in the way of treatment and preparations depends on its type. Colour influences the texture, while any skin can have a sensitive or blemished condition.

Oily skin: This is mainly due to overactive sebaceous glands and tends to affect mostly dark skin, although lighter skin may also be affected. Excess oil causes shininess, and can make the skin coarse with enlarged pores. It is prone to acne, and often gets black or whiteheads. The only consolation is that it stays younger-looking longer, has fewer wrinkles and usually improves with age. Trying to remove all oils from the skin only encourages greater gland activity, so it's important to remove only the excess oil from the surface, as too enthusiastic a treatment with harsh soap or cleansing lotion will often dehydrate the epidermis, leaving skin in a flaky condition.

Dry skin: This is due to three causes: dehydration, insufficient amount of oil secretion and ageing. Dry skin is generally of a fine texture, but looks and feels tight and drawn. It chaps, flakes and peels easily and even at an early age may show wrinkles and lines, particularly around the eyes and mouth. The best way to deal with dry skin is to try to avoid further dehydration by sealing the moisture in, or rehydration. The lack of natural oils must be compensated by rich external lubrication.

Normal or balanced skin: This type of skin exists when oil, moisture and acidity are harmonious. It is ideal but rare. This type of skin is fine-textured with no visible pores, smooth to touch and neither wet nor greasy. It has a tendency to become drier with time (ageing) so it needs care to maintain the status quo.

Combination skin: This is really skin in transition between a dry and an oily state. It gives off too much oil in the T-zone of forehead, nose and chin. The rest is dry, particularly around eyes and on cheeks. The dry and oily areas have to be treated separately.

SKIN CONDITIONS

Sensitive: This skin is usually dry and fine-textured, often with a transparent look; the upper layer being particularly thin and sensitive and likely to develop broken capillaries as in the case of rosacea. Reacts quickly to both external and internal influences – sun, wind, emotions, food, drink. Needs normal dry skincare plus extra protective, gentle lubrication. Watch for any allergies.

Blemished: Usually oily skin plus troubled with pimples. Sometimes, due to the intensity of acne, needs normal oily skincare plus attention from medicated preparations that dry and heal, and professional advice. Sometimes blemished skin develops pigmentation due to hormonal imbalances, for example during menopause.

COLOUR

The colour of the skin depends on the degree of pigmentation. Light skin tones are graded from pale to pink and beige to rosy. Dark skin tones go from olive to caramel, and brown to black. There is no basic difference in structure or quality. Dark skin generally has more sweat and sebaceous glands, so may be oilier. The sun is the great enemy of light skins, which usually have dry tendencies, so lines are created faster. The evenly distributed pigment in dark skins acts like a sun filter and its oilier surface acts as a shield, keeping moisture in. Dark skin – even black skin – can tan and burn, but less drastically than light skin. Dermatologists say that black skin is less likely to develop acne or skin cancer.

Our skin is constantly renewing itself and it takes about 30 days for a newly formed skin cell to move step by step through the layers of epidermis until it becomes cornified and stratified (hard and flat) and eventually is rubbed off the surface. Vitamin A controls the rate of cornification and anyone suffering from vitamin A deficiency will have hard, horny skin. When we apply massage oils to the top layer, the epidermis, the tiny molecules of essential oil penetrate to the dermis (or corium), where the elasticity of the skin is governed. It is in this layer that fibres of collagen, elastic fibres and fibres of connective tissues are intermingled and it is the alignment of these fibres that gives the skin its elasticity. Also in this layer are the hair roots, glands, blood vessels and lymph vessels. A complex structure indeed, which gives us the word 'complexion'.

According to doctors Robert and Elizabeth McCarter, contributing authors to *The Life Science Health System*: 'A healthy skin sings of a well-nourished body, of systemic equilibrium, of balance, of homeostasis, of sound living practices, of good inheritance, of vitality, of a clean, free flowing unobstructed bloodstream, and of organs functioning silently and efficiently in a body at peace.'

The skin is one of the first organs of the body to be affected by poor diet, vitamin and mineral deficiencies, and improper elimination. In short, it's the mirror of your health. Moist, clear radiant skin is generally a sign of good health, while skin that is dry and flaky, or oily and pimply, can be indicative of internal problems, especially where nutrition is concerned.

Remember Nature's promise: Take care of your skin and your skin will reward you with health and beauty for the rest of your life!

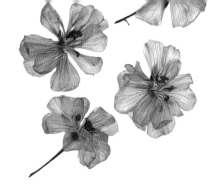

CARE OF THE SKIN

To keep your skin deep-down clean, no matter whether it's oily, combination, normal or dry, five basic practices should be observed: cleansing, toning, moisturising, high water intake and dry brushing.

1. **Cleansing:** A very important step, to be followed twice a day. Using a wash cloth or facial sponge, apply the appropriate facial cleanser for your skin type to your face and throat, and massage gently, using upward, circular strokes. This step should take about a minute, then rinse your face with clean warm water to remove all traces of the cleanser and pat dry. Aromatic cleansers are better as they do not disturb the skin's pH. Never use a harsh or strong scrub on your facial skin – always be gentle.

2. **Toning:** A toner is designed to remove any traces of cleanser that have been left behind and restore the pH balance of the skin. Herbal liquids or aromatic waters make very gentle toners: just soak a cotton ball and apply in gentle, upward strokes. No need to pat dry – go on to moisturise.

3. **Moisturising:** This is important even for oily skin. Moisturiser is designed to prevent dehydration (loss of water) of the skin. Even an oily skin can suffer from lack of water. A good moisturiser serves as a

barrier between your skin and the environment. It will help to keep the skin younger-looking for a longer time. Simply apply the appropriate moisturiser after toner, using upward, circular strokes until the moisturiser disappears. Also massage the underside of your chin to clear and activate your submandibular lymph nodes; this helps to clear toxins and restore the glow to the skin.

4. **Water intake:** Sufficient water intake is essential to maintaining soft, moist, glowing skin. It can be in almost any form, including plain water, fruit juices or raw fruit and vegetables.

5. **Dry brushing:** A MUST for smooth, clear skin. Over the course of a day, our skin eliminates more than a pound of waste through thousands of tiny sweat glands. In fact, about one-third of all the body's impurities are excreted this way. But if our pores are clogged by tight-fitting clothes, aluminium-containing synthetic antiperspirants/deodorants, or mineral-based moisturisers, there is no way for these toxic byproducts to escape, and the toxins have to seek another route to escape from the body, causing skin to look pale, pasty, pimply or diseased. So the solution is dry brushing.

As the name suggests, dry brushing is performed on *dry* skin; not oiled, not damp, but dry, before you shower. Use a natural fibre brush for gentle, not harsh, brushing over the entire body except face and breasts. Begin brushing your hands, in between the fingers, then arms, underarms, neck, chest, stomach, back, then on to each leg beginning with the feet. You'll feel wonderfully invigorated when finished and your skin will glow. Use a light aromatherapy moisturiser or herbal lotion after your shower.

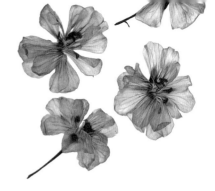

ESSENTIAL OILS AND OUR LYMPHATIC SYSTEM

The body's lymphatic system is a vitally important component in the maintenance of good health. It is a network of vessels that reach almost every part of the body. The system collects plasma and white cells that have leaked out of the blood capillaries into the spaces between the body cells. The plasma and the white cells (together called the lymph) are squeezed into the lymphatic vessels as muscles contract. Lymph returns to the blood via a vein near the heart.

Lymph nodes are converging points of various lymphatic vessels, these nodes are swellings found in the groin, armpit, neck and elsewhere. White cells in these nodes fight infection by destroying bacteria. The nodes may become enlarged if the body is actively fighting an infection.

Lymph permeates all the body tissues, removing toxins and carrying infection-fighting lymphocytes to wherever they are needed. Before toxins are excreted from the body, they must firstly pass through the lymph nodes, where they are broken down, then fed into the bloodstream, from where they pass to the organs of elimination and make their way out of the body. When essential oils enter the body through the skin, either by massage, masks, bathing or any other method, they mix with lymph and are carried along on the same journey as the toxins. During this journey, the antiseptic, antiviral, antibiotic or antifungal properties of essential oils are able to kill off harmful organisms even before they reach the lymph nodes. Because there is less infective material passing into the lymph nodes, they rarely become inflamed and are better equipped to carry out their second function, which is to produce lymphocytes.

The lymph also carries away fluids and fats from body tissues and organs – a function that prevents us from becoming obese and water-logged. Because essential oils perform an important role in keeping infection under control, the lymphatic system is able to carry off fats and fluids more easily, which means that our body shape, as well as our health, improves.

The lymphatic system is a part of the circulatory system and as such is influenced by the heart. All the body systems are interconnected, and according to the laws of acupuncture it is the lungs that govern the waterways of the body. The waterways refer to the lymphatic system, which means that as long as we are breathing, lymph is circulating around our body. It also means that any form of exercise that increases the action of the lungs is beneficial to the lymphatic system. Physical movement of the skin, such as skin brushing or massage, is also very beneficial to the free flow of lymph.

There are many health problems that may result from congested and stagnant lymph drainage. Following are some conditions that may improve with increased lymph flow:

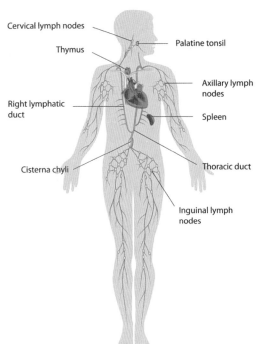

Cervical lymph nodes

Thymus

Right lymphatic duct

Cisterna chyli

Palatine tonsil

Axillary lymph nodes

Spleen

Thoracic duct

Inguinal lymph nodes

The lymphatic system.

Conditions that may improve with increased lymph flow

Arthritis	Ovarian and uterine	Headaches
Backaches	cysts	Migraines
Asthma	Fibrocystic breasts	IBS (irritable bowel
Breast cancer	Painful and enlarged	syndrome)
Cellulite	breasts	Kidney problems
Chronic fatigue	Congested lungs	Lymphoma
Prostate enlargement	Congestive heart	Lymphoedema
Psoriasis	failure	Neck and shoulder
Rheumatism	Crow's-feet	stiffness
Ringing in ears	Wrinkles	PMS
Sagging chin	Dandruff	Polyps
Sinus problems	Dizziness – vertigo	Skin disorders
Sluggishness	Earaches	Eye diseases and poor
Obesity	Oedema	vision
	Enlargement of heart	Frequent colds and flu
	Excessive tiredness	Toxin accumulation

MANUAL LYMPHATIC DRAINAGE

MLD involves light, rhythmical massage that aids the body in collecting and moving lymphatic fluid, which plays a key role in delivering nutrients, antibodies and other immune constituents to the tissue cells of the body and removing debris such as toxins, cell waste and dead particles, which are then cleansed by clusters of lymph nodes. MLD also works on the nervous system, lowering blood pressure, reducing stress and improving sleep patterns.

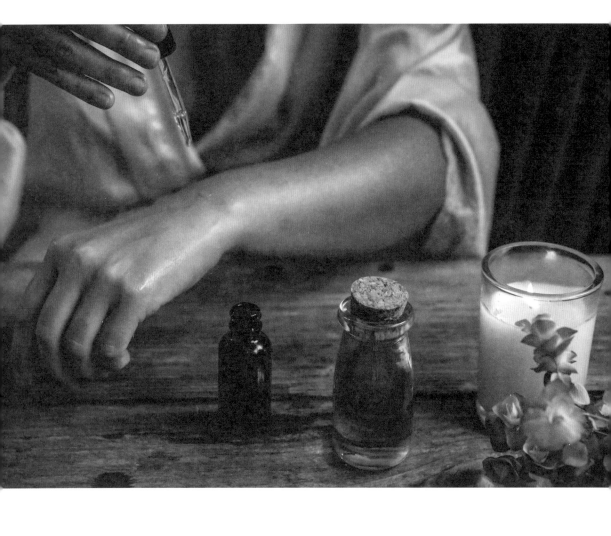

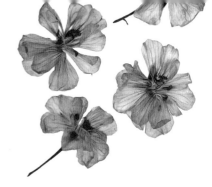

OUR BODY AND BODY PROBLEM SPOTS

The human body is a fascinating and remarkable machine. Its design is far more complex than the most advanced computer. Deep inside the body are billions of cells carrying out thousands of different functions without our conscious knowledge. The body regulates its temperature and water content, the rate of the heartbeat and numerous other processes. The coordinating centre for all these activities is the brain. It receives records and stores a greater variety of data than any computer ever could.

BODY PROBLEM SPOTS

Common external problems and problem areas in different body parts can be classified as:

The face: dry and dehydrated skin, greasy skin, open pores, blackheads and acne, acne marks, pigmentation and blemishes, maturing skin, double chins, crow's-feet, thin eyelashes, dry and chapped lips, dark circles.

Hair and head: Dry lacklustre hair, dandruff, excess grease; hair loss, tension in head, stressed-out feeling.

Back and shoulders: Congested, blemished skin, greasy skin, dull looking skin, tension in neck and shoulders.

Breasts: Sagging breasts, fibrocystic breast condition (lumps in breast), breasts too large or too small, stretch-marks, blemishes.

Upper arms, neck and elbows: Saggy upper arms, cellulite, excess fat, wrinkled elbows, rough elbows, dry skin.

Tummy and waist: Excess fat, wrinkles, stored tension in solar plexus.

Thighs and buttocks: Cellulite, obesity, stretch marks, buttocks droop, dull and lifeless skin.

Knees, ankles and feet: Fat knees, puffy knees, wrinkly knees, puffy ankles, hidden ankles, tired feet.

Hands and nails: Dry skin dehydrated skin, fat or puffy hands, brittle nails, ridged nails.

Everyone has problem spots to be worked on. So the first objective is to identify and categorise the problem spots. Take into account the age, bone structure, genetics (hereditary factors) and lifestyle of the person. If the person is big-boned, don't imagine that massage with essential oils will make them look petite.

Categorise these problem spots into major (primary), moderate (secondary) and minor (tertiary) – and make an evaluation chart (see below) so you can track progress. After listing each condition, list below them what is required to reverse the conditions. For example, if we analyse a dry, mature skin with pigmentation, we'll list them as:

	Primary condition	Secondary condition	Tertiary condition
Conditions	Dry skin	Mature/ageing	Pigmentation
Solutions	Moisturise	Rejuvenate	Regulate hormones

Then list all the essential oils which are suitable for each category and choose the best five available to you for preparing a blend.

THE FACE

The problems: Dry and dehydrated skin, greasy skin, open pores, maturing skin, lifeless skin; double-chin; pimples and pimple marks and blemishes, tired and irritated eyes, dark circles, crow's-feet, thin eyelashes, dry and chapped lips.

The causes: Lack of natural oils or excess secretion of sebum, insufficient water, smoking and lack of nourishment (inside out); polluted environment; sun, stress and hormonal imbalance.

The solutions: Massage oils to feed and nourish the skin, re-hydration of the skin with aromatic waters and rebalancing oils, cleansing and rejuvenating (face lift) massage, friction massage, facial masks and facial steaming as well as cleansing regime for the skin, decongesting oils, soothing aromatic compresses, toning the eye area, nourishing oils for lashes and brows, softening and protecting lip balms.

CARE OF THE FACE

Although there is a saying 'Don't judge a book by its cover', in reality we are often judged by the look of our face: whether we are beautiful, attractive or plain, it can be seen in our faces. The mind is mirrored in the face and when mentally stressed our face loses its attractiveness. When we feel happy and contented, a certain glow comes from within, which not only makes us feel good but is visible to others also.

Essential oils are ideally suited to skincare, for they are readily absorbed and have the ability to penetrate through to the underlying layers of the skin which are alive and active, unlike the outer dead layer of cells that are constantly being shed. Essential oils stimulate cellular regeneration, improve the circulation and help to eliminate toxins at a fundamental level. Skin that has been treated with essential oils thus becomes more dynamic and healthy. In addition, since the oils are able to travel in the bloodstream and lymphatic system, skin treatments using essential oils are vitalising to the body as a whole.

For skincare, not only the choice of correct essential oils is important, base oils are equally important. While essential oils provide the therapeutic benefits to the skin, the vegetable oils provide the nourishment. As most of the vegetable oils contain essential fatty acids (also called vitamin F) and other essential vitamins and minerals. Here's a list of important essential and carrier oils for skin and hair care:

IMPORTANT OILS FOR SKIN AND HAIR

Essential oils	Base oils
Lavender	Almond
Geranium	Olive
Frankincense	Wheatgerm
Tea-tree	Jojoba
Sandalwood	Grapeseed
Clary sage	Evening primrose
Juniper berry	Argan nut
Rosemary	Avocado
Chamomile, German & Roman	Hazelnut
Palmarosa	Rosehip seed oil
Vetiver	Macerated carrot oil
Rose	Calendula
Neroli	
Petitgrain	
Cypress	

THE MYSTERY OF PH

The natural acid/alkaline balance of healthy skin has a pH (potential hydrogen) value. If less than 7 it is acidic; if more than 7 it is alkaline. Most synthetic detergents and soaps are alkaline and can upset the natural acid mantle which protects against germs, dirt and invasive bacteria. It is therefore important that you do not strip the skin of this protective mantle and only use substances like essential oils which have neutral pH value (between 6.5–7).

OILY OR GREASY SKIN

Greasy skin is only a problem after the onset of puberty and before this turning point in our lives, the majority of us have smooth skin. At birth we have approximately 100 sebaceous (oil producing) glands on every square centimetre of our skin with the exception of the soles of our feet, palms of our hands and the eardrums, but immediately after birth these glands are much more intense – up to 900 per square centimetre on the face, scalp, forehead and genital region.

Our sebaceous glands produce a thick, oily colourless secretion produced in cells or lobes, which break down and empty their contents in ducts, which in turn empty into follicles. The lifespan of each one of these lobes is only about a week, but it is an ongoing process that lubricates the skin continually.

The composition of sebum is complex. It is a mix of hundreds of fatty acids – a significant proportion of them being the fatty acids palmitic, myristic, stearic, oleic and linoleic. It is the secretion of sebum onto the skin of the face and scalp that can become a problem for teenagers and older women as the face looks shiny, make-up runs, the presence of surface oil can cause clogged pores, which are open to the air (blackheads) or closed (whiteheads), and infection of the ducts by microorganisms can produce pimples.

Thorough cleansing of the skin is of vital importance: Cleansing must not strip the skin of its protective mantle, which maintains the natural pH balance. Carried out several times a day using aromatic waters (gels), cleansing will prevent a buildup of sebum on the skin's surface. Facial steaming and the use of clay masks can be very helpful in keeping the complexion clear and blemish-free, and should include one of the following essential oils: lemon, geranium, lavender, bergamot (FCF), juniper berry, petitgrain, neroli and rosemary.

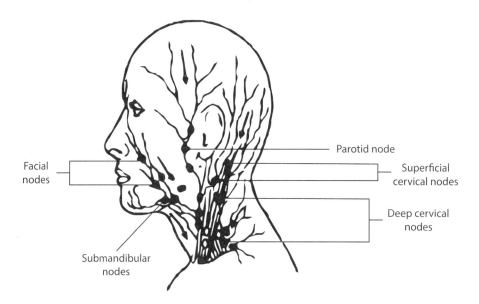

Cleansing: Cleansing with aromatic waters (gels) and using an aromatic facial steam bring the skin into contact with a very small amount of essential oil, which has beneficial results, but to treat a blemished complexion, it is necessary to apply a stronger concentration of essential oils in a light fatty oil base. The reason to use a fatty oil on an already greasy skin is firstly not all fatty oils are especially greasy, and secondly essential oils need to be diluted before application to the skin. As essential oils dissolve in fatty acids, the preferred medium is fatty oil. Fatty oils contain acids in much the same way as the skin and we know that essential oils dissolve into the oil secreted by the sebaceous glands. When an essential oil such as lavender is massaged into the face, its antiseptic properties seep down into the deep layers of the skin to kill the bacteria, thus protecting and healing the skin and preventing infection.

- A simple recipe for a nightly cleansing massage is 2 drops of a blend of lavender, geranium, petitgrain, juniper berry and frankincese oils plus 1 teaspoon (5 ml) of a good quality light fatty oil such as grapeseed. Take care to remove all the traces of the oil from the face with a tissue or with cottonwool. Or:

- Add 3 drops each of lemon, rosemary, petitgrain and lavender to 2 tablespoons (30 ml) of light carrier oil such as grapeseed, sweet almond or olive with avocado (for penetration). Massage gently all over and remove all the traces of the oil from the face with a moist cotton swab, you'll be able to see all the dirt and grime.

- A good toner/cleanser for greasy or combination skin is to mix 5 drops each of petitgrain, juniper, lavender and geranium with 25 ml of vodka and 75 ml of orange flower water/rosewater. Let it stand for up to a month then filter. Use it for facial cleansing twice daily.

- After thorough cleansing you can **nourish and moisturise** the face with a rejuvenating massage oil containing any three to five essential oils including lavender, frankincense, geranium, sandalwood, Roman chamomile or juniper berry, to a total of 15 drops in 30 ml (2 tablespoons) of nourishing base oil, such as jojoba, sweet almond, evening primrose or wheatgerm. You can also make a combination of base oils to make your formulation more effective. This nourishing combination can be used once or twice daily, preferably on moist skin after washing.

- Spotty and greasy skins will benefit most from a **facial steam** once or twice a week incorporating a healing, antiseptic essential oil such as tea-tree, geranium, juniper berry or lavender (just 3–5 drops in a bowl of steaming hot water). Young problem skins also benefit from a facial steam once or twice a week, alternating with a face mask on other nights.
- An excellent basic **purifying and rejuvenating face mask** for greasy skin can be made by mixing 2 tablespoons of green clay, 2 tablespoons of cornflour, 1 egg yolk and 1 teaspoon of evening primrose oil with 1 drop each of rosemary and lavender. Leave on the skin for 15 minutes then rinse off with cool water.

DRY AND DEHYDRATED SKIN

Dry skin becomes wrinkled more easily than greasy skin and needs to be moisturised regularly, especially when exposed to the effects of the environment and climate (too cold or too much sun).

There are many essential oils which, when blended together and incorporated into a fatty base oil, make wonderful massage oils. We can create a blend to feed, regularise, moisturise and rejuvenate ageing skin or bring antiseptic healing powers to troubled skin.

- A good **toner/cleanser** for dry skin can be made by adding 5 drops each of lemon, lavender, petitgrain and geranium to 100 ml rosewater, letting it stand for up to a month before filtering.
- **Facial steaming** is also beneficial for dry skin, incorporating healing, antiseptic essential oils such as sandalwood or lavender (just 3 drops in a bowl of hot water) once a fortnight, to be followed with moisturiser.
- A **moisturising treatment for dry skin** can be made by adding 5 drops each of lavender, geranium and sandalwood to 75 ml of rosewater, letting it stand for up to a month before filtering. Then

add 25 ml of glycerine and shake well. To be used twice daily.

- For **moisturising dry sensitive skin,** it is important to avoid all possible irritants and to use only the gentlest oils: Roman chamomile, lavender, sandalwood, vetiver and geranium or rose are the best choice. Add 7–8 drops of any of the above oils or a combination of 3–5 oils to 1 tablespoon (15 ml) of a combination of jojoba, sweet almond or argan nut oil.
- An excellent basic **purifying and rejuvenating face mask** for dry and sensitive skin can made by mixing 2 tablespoons of green clay, 2 teaspoons of cornflour, 1 egg yolk and 1 teaspoon of avocado or almond oil with 1 drop each of geranium and sandalwood. Leave on the skin for 15 minutes then rinse off with cool water.

AGEING SKIN, THREAD VEINS AND WRINKLES

There are two kinds of ageing: one is intrinsic or chronological ageing, which is inevitable because of our body's cells' potential for multiplying, but limited life expectancy. The body's own mechanisms control this, such as hormones, growth factors and vitamins. Day-to-day physical, mental and emotional stresses also play a major role. Just as night follows day, the passage of time means that it is inevitable that we will get older.

Extrinsic ageing is mainly due to environmental factors like excess exposure to the sun. It is also called photo intrinsic or active ageing. Lifestyle also affects ageing.

As the skin gets older, cell division slows down and the skin becomes drier because of the reduced activity of the skin's oil glands. The slowing down of cell division means that the various organs in the skin work less efficiently. The inner dermis network of collagen and elastic fibres that give the skin its plain contours, suppleness and firmness begins to alter, losing its tension and plumpness, and wrinkles form. The outer layer of skin cells, the epidermis, also becomes thinner, resulting in the flat, lifeless appearance of older skin.

Nothing can stop this natural process, but massage with essential oils can do more than most potions to slow down the effects. Essential oils encourage the skin cells to regenerate more efficiently and help the skin to lubricate itself, keeping it supple and less prone to wrinkling.

- Regular use of a facial oil containing cytophylactic oils (those that stimulate new cell growth and prevent wrinkles) is vital. They are lavender, geranium, neroli, frankincense, sandalwood, Roman chamomile, rose, vetiver and palmarosa. Add 7–8 drops of the combination of any three of these oils to 1 tablespoon (15 ml) of jojoba or wheatgerm oil, for gentle application, especially to the area around the eyes before retiring.

- A good basic blend for the face and neck is 1 tablespoon (15 ml) jojoba oil, 1 teaspoon (5 ml) wheatgerm oil, 1 tablespoon (15 ml) of grapeseed oil, to which you add 6 drops of lavender, 4 drops of geranium, 3 drops of frankincense and 2 drops of sandalwood oil.

- Thread veins and broken capillaries are best treated using the aforesaid facial oil with the addition of 1 drop of Roman chamomile or rose oil.

- A face mask made by mixing 2 tablespoons of green clay, 2 teaspoons of runny honey, 1 teaspoon of water and 4 drops of rose or geranium oil, used once a week, helps rejuvenation. You may also add 2 drops of lavender and 1 drop of frankincense to enhance the effect.

FRICTION MASSAGE FOR REJUVENATION

Most beauticians insist that facial massage should be of lightest possible strokes for fear of stretching the delicate tissues of the skin. It's true in the case of sensitive skin, acne, or skin with broken veins –i n these cases, the skin should be handled with gentle care. But in the case of normal, dry or ageing skin, friction massage with selected essential oil blends has many benefits. It tones the underlying muscles, keeping them in good shape.

It nourishes the skin by bringing blood to the surface, thereby allowing dietary nutrients available for cell renewal. It also rubs away dead skin cells, helping to make the complexion look lighter and more youthful. Massage the face with upward and outward motions towards the ears. It is also important to massage the underside of the chin area to clear the submandibular lymph nodes. The best way to do this is: holding two fingers like a V, place one finger in the front of the ear and the other behind the ear and draw the hand with gentle pressure all along the chin to the other side of the ear, then repeat the action at the other ear.

Secure hair back from forehead and apply the massage oil blend from the hairline to the chin, working on one section of the face at a time. Tense the muscles (as a man does when shaving) so that the skin is not stretched. Starting with one section (say, the left cheek), press and rotate the skin and underlying muscles using the first three fingers of the left hand. Feel for any sore areas, and gently but firmly massage those areas until the skin begins to feel hot. Next, put your right thumb inside your mouth so that the pad of the thumb is pressing against the inside of the cheek. Squeeze the flesh between thumb and fingers and move the thumb in tiny circular movements so that all the flesh inside the cheek has been massaged. Repeat the movements on the right side of the face. Next, place the palms of your hands on the cheeks and, with facial muscles tensed, buff the cheeks with circular movements. Massage of the forehead follows; in order to tense the muscles, simply close the eyes tightly and then to buff the skin with the palm of the hand. Begin in the centre of the forehead and with a circular motion work outwards towards the temples. Before massaging the chin, bring the lips together so that they are not visible (as a woman does to spread lipstick evenly after application) and with the palms of the hands buff the skin. Move the mouth (again as a man does while shaving) so that there is enough muscle tension and massage in this way around to the mouth, so that tiny lines are encouraged to disappear.

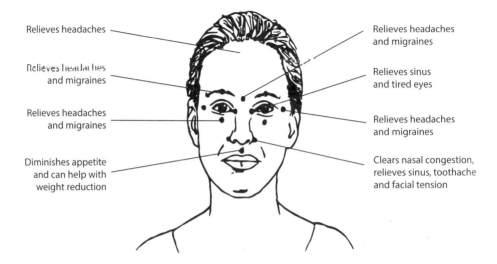

Relieves headaches

Relieves headaches and migraines

Relieves headaches and migraines

Diminishes appetite and can help with weight reduction

Relieves headaches and migraines

Relieves sinus and tired eyes

Relieves headaches and migraines

Clears nasal congestion, relieves sinus, toothache and facial tension

DOUBLE CHIN

A double chin can be greatly helped by massaging the skin with the following blend:

To a 30 ml bottle add:

- 3 drops lemongrass oil
- 3 drops grapefruit oil
- 3 drops lavender oil
- 3 drops cypress oil
- 3 drops orange oil
- 15 ml jojoba or argan oil
- 15 ml grapeseed oil

Though lemongrass is very powerful and not normally used on the face as it can irritate the delicate skin, it has a remarkable ability to decongest the tissues by burning up toxins in the connective tissue. The chin is an area where fat can accumulate easily and where toxins can lodge.

Apply the above blend to the underside of the chin and tilt the head back so that the skin of the neck is taut. Using only the tips of the first two fingers of each hand, slide the fingertips along the jawline until they reach the angle of the jaw. Repeat several times. Position the same fingers under the jawbone in the centre of the chin and gently stroke the 'double chin', drawing the fingers down the neck towards the cervical lymph nodes. Continue this gentle stroking of the under-chin area and be sensitive to any lumps and bumps that may be under the skin's surface. Gently massage these toxic and stagnant spots to encourage them to disperse and immediately after working on this area, spend a few moments massaging the lymph nodes involved with the drainage of fats and toxins from the head and neck.

If the skin under the chin is loose and saggy, replace the lemongrass oil in this blend with vetiver and cypress oils and massage the area, as vetiver oil has the ability to attract and retain moisture in the underlying tissues of the skin, making the flesh look plumper, while cypress will tighten the skin.

ACNE (PIMPLES OR SPOTS)

Acne is a condition in which the skin of the face and sometimes at the neck, shoulders, chest and back is covered to a greater or lesser extent with pimples, blackheads, whiteheads and boils. Acne usually results from a hormonal imbalance or an incorrect diet or both, being the factors that affect the production of sebum. Sometimes acne is the result of dandruff; in this case acne spots are more on the forehead and the back.

A variety of factors including too-frequent washing, an unhealthy diet, hormonal imbalance and stress may affect the production of sebum and sweat, causing too much or too little to be secreted, with consequently greasy or dry skin. The typical onset of acne in adolescence is related to the increased activity of the glands, including the sebaceous glands. Most of the oil gets into pores; when the surface pores are clogged with sebaceous gland secretions and keratin, and so much extra oil is being secreted that it backs up into the ducts, the result is the formation of skin blemishes, characteristic of acne. In the case of acne due to hormonal disturbance, taking 1 teaspoon (5 ml) of evening primrose oil orally on a daily basis for 3 months helps a great deal.

The blackheads are dark not because they are dirty but because the fatty material in the clogged pore is oxidised and discoloured by the air that reaches it. If this substance is infected by bacteria, it turns into a pimple. Pimples should not be picked or squeezed, because the pressure can rupture the surrounding membrane and spread the infection further.

Treatment

Lifestyle: Gentle ultraviolet rays can greatly relieve acne, so take every opportunity you can to go out in the sun (but do not overexpose the skin).
Diet: Follow a healthy balanced diet, avoiding spicy and fatty foods, in particular dairy products. The diet should include plenty of other sources of protein and calcium-rich food. Eat plenty of fresh fruits and green vegetables. Drink up to 2 litres of water daily.
Essential oils: Those that regulate sebum production and purify the blood include juniper berry, lemon, cypress and geranium. Tea-tree, lavender, palmarosa and geranium are antiseptic and healing, while German chamomile and petitgrain help to reduce inflammation.

- Apply an aromatic flower water as a toner/cleanser to the skin, morning and evening. To prepare, mix 25 ml of cider vinegar and 75 ml of rosewater with 5 drops each of lemon, geranium, tea-tree and lavender. Let it mature for up to a month, and then filter before use with coffee filter paper. (It is better to make a batch in one go only.)
- Use a light facial oil containing 2 teaspoons of grapeseed oil, 1 teaspoon of argan nut oil and 1 teaspoon of jojoba oil, and add 3 drops each of tea-tree, juniper, geranium and lavender. Apply gently every night on moist skin after washing the face. This will also help

clearing acne scars.

- Individual pimples can be dabbed with neat lavender and tea-tree (check sensitisation first).

- A good facial mask can be made by mixing 2 tablespoons of green clay or kaolin and 2 teaspoon of yoghurt or rosewater with 2 drops each of juniper, geranium and cypress.

- To unclog the pores of the skin, put 3 drops each of petitgrain and geranium in a bowl of steaming water as facial steam. Putting pine needle oil mixed with water on the stove when having a sauna has a similar effect on the whole body.

Emergency pimple treatment

Pimples should never be squeezed when they are small red bumps, because at this stage there is nothing to remove and result is only bruising of the tissues. However, when a pimple has come to a head, you have a choice of whether to dab it with neat lavender and tea-tree or in an emergency (such as an important social occasion) you can squeeze the spot. Though this is not recommended, if carried out carefully you can get rid of the waste material and whitehead in the pimple.

A sharp needle should be sterilised by first wiping with a piece of cottonwool moistened with 1 drop of lavender. Gently prick the spot with the needle – not downward into the spot but sideways, so that the tip of the needle is parallel with the face. With clean cottonwool, apply sufficient pressure to discharge the accumulated debris (a mixture of bacteria and dead lymph cells) and finally dab the area with one of the antiseptic oils such as lavender, tea-tree, juniper, lemon, palmarosa or geranium. This may sting for a few seconds but it will prevent the spread of infection. Use no make up for 24 hours.

An alternate to squeezing is to take facial steam at the first signs of a spot. The hot moist vapours combined with antiseptic and healing aromas promote elimination through the skin and help to unblock the clogged pores – often the cause of blackheads and spots (pimples).

THE EYES

It is said that the eyes are the windows to the soul. The eyes are our most expressive features and should be cared for. The best eye treatment of all is a good night's sleep, but the kind of lifestyle we all have – late nights, looking at mobile phones and TV/computer screens most of the time, spending time around smokers or in polluted air, allergies, not removing mascara, make up remover going in the eyes – results in our 'windows' looking puffy, bloodshot, irritated or having dark circles beneath them. They may even sting and water.

For a night-time eye moisturiser: On a damp, freshly cleansed face apply a few drops of jojoba, grapeseed, sweet almond or evening primrose oil and mix together with your ring finger, then gently pat the oil around (not directly on) the eye, beginnng at the outer corner and slowly moving beneath your eye towards the inner corner, then onto the very upper portion of the lid and back out to the outer corner.

Do this several times, then blot off any excess oil. Try to leave a thin film of oil on the skin. The oil should not be applied directly on the lids and lashes. If the oil gets into the eye, it could clog the tear ducts and cause puffiness (which we are trying to avoid). The delicate eye area will draw the moisture it needs from the surrounding moisturised tissue.

You can also use an aromatic eye compress using lavender water (prepare by adding 10 drops lavender oil to 200 ml of spring water and shaking well) to soothe irritated, puffy eyes. Saturate a piece of cotton pad with lavender aromatic water, then remove excess by squeezing before applying the pad to the eyes. Lie down for at least 10 minutes while the compress is in place. An alternative to this compress is thin slices of cold cucumber or potato.

Crow's-feet: To treat wrinkles of the delicate skin around the eye and tighten the skin, apply an egg white face mask with rose or geranium oil. Whisk the egg white in a small bowl and when frothy add 2 drops of rose or geranium oil. Mix for a few seconds more and apply to the skin immediately around the eye socket. The upper eyelids and eyebrows may be included in this tightening mask. Allow to dry and rinse off with wet cotton pads. While the skin is still damp, apply a little wheatgerm oil and jojoba oil blend and gently pat into the skin at the outer edges of the eyes.

Conjunctivitis: Conjunctivitis is the inflammation of the conjunctiva, a thin, delicate membrane that covers the eyeball and lines the eyelid. Conjunctivitis is an extremely common eye problem because the conjunctiva is continually exposed to microorganisms and environmental agents that can cause infections or allergic reactions. Essential oils help to prevent and treat conjuntivitis. Simply soak a cottonwool ball in water and put a drop or two of a combination of tea-tree, lavender and Roman chamomile. Close the eyes and put the cotton ball on your eyes; leave on the eyes for 5–10 minutes. Repeat 3 times a day and your conjunctivitis will be relieved in a day or two.

Thin eyelashes and eyebrows: When eyelashes become thin because of the constant wearing of mascara, they should be given a holiday from mascara and instead be treated with a coating of jojoba oil. Apply this blend with a mascara applicator and also massage a little on to the eyelids where the lashes spring forth. The skin surrounding the eye is very sensitive and feeding the eyelashes should not be repeated too frequently. Application once a week is ample.

The condition of especially thin and straggly eyebrows can also be improved by rubbing a little jojoba oil along their length.

Lips: Our lips, unlike the rest of our skin, do not contain any sebaceous glands (oil glands) or sweat glands to keep them moisturised and lubricated. The lipsticks used on the lips should not only beautify but also prevent them from drying and cracking, however, many lipstick brands tend to dry out, which can make the lips flake and peel and look unsightly.

Dry lips may also occur when we are unavoidably outside on a windy day or when we have had too much sun on our face. However, dry lips also indicate that we are not drinking enough water. Make this protective lip balm to protect dry, chapped lips:

This protective lip balm for dry/chapped lips can also double as cuticle cream. It is good for everyone, even children.

Preparation time: 20–30 minutes

- 5 teaspoons (25 ml) jojoba oil
- 1 teaspoon (5 ml) avocado oil
- 5 drops each of geranium, lavender and sandalwood essential oils
- Mix all together. Store in a small glass jar. Makes approximately 30 ml.

HEAD AND HAIR CARE

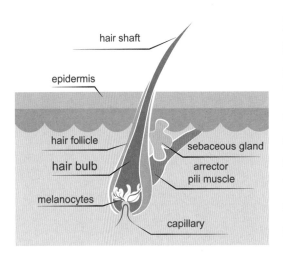

The problems: Dry lacklustre hair, brittle hair, excess grease, hair loss, tension in the head, feeling stressed out, and dandruff.

The causes: Lack of nourishment, external chemicals (hair dyes and perms), environment, sun, hormonal imbalance, mental and emotional stress.

The solutions: Aromatic oils for hair treatment, hair shampoos and rinses, head and neck massage.

HEALTHY HAIR

Our hair is only a collection of individual hairs – approximately 250,000 – each one deep-rooted in the scalp and just as dependent on good nutrition as the skin or any other part of our body. Hair originates in tiny sacs or follicles deep in the dermis layer of the skin tissue. The part of the hair below the skin's surface is the root; the part above is the shaft. Hair follicles are closely connected to the sebaceous glands, which secrete oil to the scalp and give hair its natural sheen. Hair grows at the rate of 1 centimetre per month, although some people's hair grows faster or slower than average. Healthy hair growth depends a lot on the diet: a healthy diet leads to healthy hair.

Hair is a complex cellular structure. Each strand, no matter how fine it may look, consists of three layers. The outer layer, or cuticle, is made up of overlapping scales that protect the inner layers. The next layer, or the cortex, is made up of long thin cells and is the most important, for it gives the hair its elastic resilience and contains the pigment, which provides the colouring. The innermost layer, or medulla, is spongy tissue and the cells sometimes contain granules of colour pigment.

The part of the hair visible above the skin is the shaft and the part beneath is the root. The root is not a single entity, as it is enclosed in a sac called the hair follicle, and at the base of this is a tiny hair nodule called the papilla, which is the storehouse for the nourishment of the hair strand. Interlinked to the follicles are sacs containing sebum which lubricate the hair and give it gloss and suppleness. An underactive or blocked sebaceous gland means dry hair; an overactive one means oily hair.

We are inclined to forget that healthy hair is a part of a healthy body, and directly affected by physical metabolism and emotional balance. Its texture may be determined by genes but its strength and condition are determined by what it is fed. A high-protein diet with lots of fresh fruits and vegetables is good for hair. Foods containing vitamins of the B complex are essential.

Also important are vitamins A and C. The minerals iron, iodine and copper are the most beneficial. Lack of iodine can be most detrimental.

Like skin, hair can be dry, oily or balanced. The wonderful washablilty of hair is one of its main assets. The ritual of washing is the first and basic beauty routine for all hair types. Oily hair requires washing every 2 to 3 days, while dry hair can be washed every 5 to 7 days. The modern rule is wash often, wash lightly and use shampoo sparingly.

Sometimes, even if our diet is sensible and nutritious, we may not benefit from the nutrients if our body is not absorbing enough vitamins and minerals from what we have eaten. Stress is one common reason why we sometimes fail to absorb sufficient goodness from our food. This is why, when someone is suffering badly from stress, their hair can start thinning and their skin may look as though they have suddenly 'aged'. Natural hair loss is between 50–100 hairs per day; more than that is considered abnormal.

Topically, there is much we can do to improve the condition of the scalp – the flowerbed or soil from which the hair blossoms. And just as we must feed the soil if we wish to produce beautiful roses, so it is with our scalp. Essential oils, when massaged into the scalp, will penetrate through the epidermis to the dermis and connective tissue where the hair bulb is rooted.

USEFUL OILS

The perfect combination of external nutrients for the scalp and hair are the aromatherapy essential and base oils. Rosemary and ylang ylang stimulate the scalp, and ylang ylang and cedarwood are balancing oils that help to prevent further hair loss. Jojoba and argan nut oils protect and contribute greatly to the process of cell renewal, and therefore are recommended as base oils. Sweet almond is considered as a tonic for the scalp for all types of hair.

HEAD AND HAIR TREATMENT

Massaging the head

A gentle nightly massage of the scalp will relieve any tightness caused by stress. When stressed, our muscles tense up causing, among other problems, headaches and nausea. But beyond the noticeable physical symptoms, tension is also responsible for preventing the normal circulation of blood and lymph, sebum and other nutrients. In effect, if we are really stressed out, we can literally be starving our hair to death. Massaging the head will dispel tension caused by stress, whether emotional, mental or environmental, by relaxing the scalp and allowing the circulation of blood, lymph and sebum. Essential oils diluted in jojoba or argan nut oil are used for the purpose of massage, enhancing the effect of massage by providing external nutrients and thereby helping to prevent hair loss and improving the health of the scalp. Choose any of the following formulations according to hair type:

For dry, lacklustre hair	For excess grease	For normal hair
2 drops of rosemary oil	2 drops of juniper oil	2 drops of palmarosa oil
2 drops of lavender oil	2 drops of lemon oil	2 drops of lemon oil
2 drops of cedarwood oil	2 drops of rosemary oil	2 drops of rosemary oil
2 drops of patchouli oil	2 drops of cedarwood oil	2 drops of ylang ylang oil
4 teaspoons of jojoba/ argan nut oil	2 teaspoons jojoba/ argan nut oil	2 teaspoons of jojoba/ argan nut oil
1 teaspoon of wheatgerm oil	3 teaspoons of grapeseed oil	3 teaspoons of sesame oil

- A few drops (approximately 1%) of an essential oil suited to your hair type can be added to your shampoo – it is always better to use a mild or pH-neutral shampoo that does not strip the hair of its protective acid mantle. For greasy hair, use rosemary and lemon, for dry hair, patchouli or cedarwood, for normal dark hair, rosemary and ylang ylang oil.
- A good rinse for all hair types is to add 5 drops of rosemary or ylang ylang essential oils to 1 tablespoon of cider vinegar, using it for the final rinse. It will also help to remove soap/shampoo chemicals residue and restore the pH balance of the scalp.

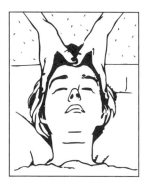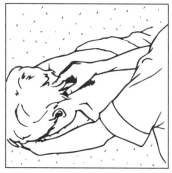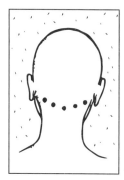

Head massage pressure points.

DANDRUFF

Dandruff may take the form of fine, dry powdery flakes or coarse, waxy scales that stick to the hair and scalp, causing intense irritation. With the latter type of dandruff, resist the temptation to scratch your head since this may cause bleeding and infection. In case the facial skin becomes oily and pimples/spots develop on forehead, wash hair frequently and choose a hairstyle that keeps the hair off the forehead. Sometimes this condition can be confused with either eczema or psoriasis of the scalp, so it is important to obtain an accurate diagnosis from a trichologist.

Treatment

Lifestyle and diet: In the case of oily dandruff, wash your hair frequently using a mild shampoo. Get plenty of exercise outdoors in the fresh air, and avoid spicy food and dairy products. Dry dandruff is often stress related. Choose one of the following according to type:

For dry flaking scalps	For oily scaly scalps
3 drops of lavender	5 drops of Atlas cedarwood oil
3 drops of geranium oil	5 drops of rosemary oil
6 drops of rosemary oil	5 drops of lemon oil
3 drops tea-tree oil	5 drops of juniper berry oil
4 drops cedarwood oil	5–6 teaspoons of carrier oil,
5–6 teaspoons of carrier oil	vodka or water

These blends should be massaged into the scalp and left for two hours or overnight. Shampoo and rinse thoroughly. Make up the final rinse by adding the same blend of essential oils to a jug of water. Stir well before using. Repeat treatment every alternate day, decreasing to twice a week.

THE BREASTS

The problems: Sagging breasts, fibrocystic (lumpy) breasts, too large or too small, stretch marks and blemishes, breast cancer.

The causes: Loss of elasticity, gravity, genetics. Poor circulation, hormonal imbalances, rapid weight gain or loss.

The solutions: Skin brushing while bathing, massage and chest packs.

The breasts are the ultimate symbol of womanly beauty, although no more than a mass of adipose tissue until hormonally changed into a milk-producing machine. Despite being coveted objects of adornment, the breasts are often neglected in terms of physical care, merely to be crammed into bras, basques and bodies – completely taken for granted. Like the rest of the body, the breasts contain connective tissues which siphon off toxins and infections, and muscle fibre, which can be damaged either by being stretched or by being constantly under tension. Massage of the breasts with aromatic oils can help to keep the breasts not only in good shape but also in good health too.

FIBROCYSTIC BREASTS

Fibrocystic breast condition, also called mastalgia, is characterised by lumpiness with pain and tenderness that fluctuate with the menstrual cycle. Many breast lumps are due to fibrocystic changes. The lumps can be caused by a collection of fibrous tissue in an area of the breast. The condition is very common and benign, especially in the 30–50 year age group. Fibrocystic breasts are not malignant (cancerous) and the condition tends to resolve; in some cases, after menopause.

What causes fibrocystic breasts?
Fibrocystic breast condition involves the glandular breast tissue. Occupying a major portion of the breast, the glandular tissue is surrounded by fatty tissue and support elements.

The most significant cause of fibrocystic breast condition is a woman's normal hormonal changes during her menstrual cycle, as this condition mostly occurs in women of child-bearing age. During the process of hormonal changes, when the body is preparing for ovulation, a possible pregnancy, it secretes oestrogen and progesterone. These hormones cause cells in the uterus lining and breast tissue to grow and multiply. In the breast, oestrogen and progesterone stimulate the growth of breast glandular tissue and increase the activity of blood vessels, cell metabolism and supporting tissue. All this activity may contribute to the feeling of breast fullness and fluid retention that women commonly experience before their menstrual period.

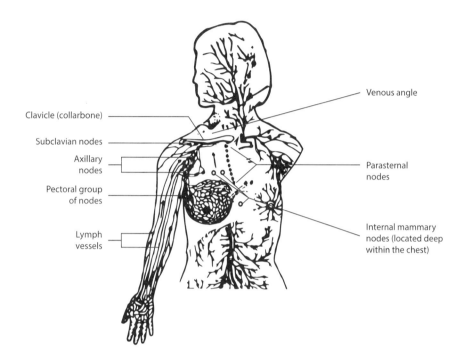

Clavicle (collarbone)

Subclavian nodes

Axillary nodes

Pectoral group of nodes

Lymph vessels

Venous angle

Parasternal nodes

Internal mammary nodes (located deep within the chest)

If pregnancy does not occur, the uterine lining is discarded and passes out of the body during menstruation. However, the stimulated breast cells cannot just be discarded. Instead, many undergo apoptosis, programmed self-destruction or 'cell suicide'. During this process of cell breakdown, inflammation and debris may lead to scarring, or fibrosis, that may damage glandular tissue within the breast. Fibrocystic breast condition seems to result from the cumulative effect of repeated monthly hormonal cycles, starting with puberty.

From my experience of healing work, I have observed that our blocked emotions affect two of our chakras in particular – sacral and heart. In the case of sacral chakra blockage due to emotional issues, lymphatics (primarily inguinal nodes) may get blocked and become sore, affecting ovulation, the menstrual cycle (irregular or painful), and sometimes leading to uterine fibroids. When the heart chakra is blocked because of painful emotions such as anguish, it affects the axillary nodes and circulation around the breast area, so can also be one of the causes for fibrocystic breast condition.

Treatment for fibrocystic breast condition

I have observed positive results on breast lumps by aromatherapy oil massage using circular movements towards the armpits to the axillary nodes. Ingestion of evening primrose oil is also very helpful. The recommended dosage is 1 teaspoon (5 mm) of pure evening primrose oil, initially for 3 to 6 months. (See Appendix 1, page 325.) Recommended essential oils are juniper berry, rose or geranium, clary sage and fennel seed oils. You can use 4 drops of each of these oils in 2 tablespoons (30 ml) of a good base oil. To be massaged twice daily all around the breast termination in the armpits.

SAGGING BREASTS WITH STRETCH MARKS

When there is a sudden weight gain or loss, the skin sometimes scars, leaving a constant reminder of weight change in the form of tiny silver lines. Stretch marks won't vanish in a few weeks as it takes far longer than that for new skin to grow, but it is possible to reduce the visible scarring over a period of time. Just by massaging the breasts with a suitable essential oil blend and by increasing the elasticity of the skin, the effect of the stretch marks will lessen and the breast tone will improve.

Skin brushing

As a measure of self-help to take care of the breasts, skin brushing once a week is important. For skin brushing, take a nailbrush and, without using much pressure, run the bristles from the breast bone out to the armpit. Brush across the entire breast, always in the direction of the armpits where the axillary lymph nodes are housed. Lifting up one arm, brush the underside of the upper arm towards the armpit and then brush the armpit itself. Underneath this area of skin, which has made a huge amount of money for the perfume and deodorant industry, lies a cluster of lymph nodes, vitally placed to drain lymph from the arms and breasts (see figure, page 214), You can even use your hand to massage yourself every day while taking your shower and when you remove your bra. Use your knuckles to knead the area of armpits to decongest the axillary nodes.

Massaging the breasts

The massage techniques are the same for every woman: circular movements towards the armpits. The only difference is the blend of the oils used. For regular massage the following blend is most suitable:

Breast massage blend

2 drops of geranium oil

2 drops of lavender oil

1 drop of vetiver oil

1 drop of cypress oil

Add to 4 teaspoons (20 ml) of a suitable carrier oil, or mix of oils (such as 1 teaspoon each of avocado, wheatgerm, grapeseed, and jojoba or argan nut oils).

For women who feel their breasts are too small and would like to try to increase their size, the following blend is most suitable:

Blend for small breasts

2 drops of geranium oil

3 drops of vetiver oil

2 drops of lavender oil

2 drops of clary sage oil

Add to 4 teaspoons (20 ml) of a suitable carrier oil, or mix of oils (such as 1 teaspoon each of avocado, wheatgerm, grapeseed, and jojoba or argan nut oils).

Whichever blend is chosen, and whether or not a change in size is achieved, massage oil will definitely improve the muscle tone of the breasts and perk up sagging breasts. The feel of skin will become silky and smooth, and the general health of the breasts will improve.

During the massage the lymph nodes get massaged, taking away toxins and dead matter from the mammary glands and bring a fresh supply of lymph containing lymphocytes to recognise and kill unwanted organisms such as bacteria and viruses, boosting the immune system.

Chest pack

Sometimes the skin in the centre of the chest (from just above the cleavage to the base of the neck) becomes spotty, which is the last thing wanted by anybody. Just as a face pack constantly refreshes and revitalises the skin, so does a chest pack. Use after a breast massage.

2 tablespoons of green clay

2 tablespoons of kaolin

2 teaspoons of water

2 drops of myrtle oil or geranium oil

Add 1 teaspoon of jojoba oil and mix in, then spread across the chest. After applying the pack, it is advisable to lie down for approximately 15 minutes while the clay dries. Cover chest with a hand towel before getting up to clean to avoid dry clay flaking off. After cleaning, pat dry.

BACK AND SHOULDERS

The problems: Congested skin dotted with pimples, greasy skin with open pores, dull-looking skin, tension in the upper back and neck, stiffness in the shoulders.

The causes: Lack of movement (of skin and muscles), stagnation, emotional/mental stress, lack of air, improper diet, dehydration.

The solutions: Aromatic baths (cleaning with friction strip), skin brushing, back compress with body wrap, massage.

All the above problems respond to bathing with aromatic oil, friction and skin brushing. Some of them, such as congested skin, greasy skin and dull looking skin, can be treated by a body wrap or back pack. For stiffness and tension in the neck and shoulders, the best treatment is massage starting from the centre of the neck, with gentle kneading, followed by massage and lymphatic drainage towards the armpits.

Pimples or spots on the back are due to bacterial infection, mostly a result of dandruff. Since all the essential oils are bactericidal, their use in any form, whether in a bath, compress, massage oil or body wrap is very effective in tackling the condition.

An aromatic bath for the shoulders

Congested skin on the back can be stimulated and improved considerably by taking an aromatic bath with 6–10 drops of lavender, juniper, geranium or rosemary, or a combination of all. Alternatively, a blend of 3 drops of lavender, 2 drops of juniper and 3 drops of rosemary can be used.

For **greasy skin,** the most suitable oils are lemon, juniper berry, lavender, rosemary, geranium, and petitgrain.

For **dry skin,** suitable oils are sandalwood, patchouli, lavender, geranium or frankincense.

Skin brushing

Like bathing, skin brushing helps the skin eliminate unwanted materials and toxins; just run the bristles of a loofah or brush along the upper arm from elbow to shoulder and from the crease of the elbow to the armpit, until the entire skin surface is covered. Then brush across the shoulders and behind the neck up to the collarbone. Under the collarbone is a collection of lymph nodes that drain impurities away from the upper chest and neck. Women are particularly vulnerable to congestion around the shoulders because of the bra they may wear for many hours a day, which will definitely cause a certain amount of pressure; even slight pressure endured for a protracted period of time will have a negative effect.

Friction rub

The back is an ideal site for elimination of the body's toxins and waste products. A spotty back with white or blackheads can be caused by a build-up of sweat and sebum which has not been cleaned thoroughly.

The skin of the back can be scrubbed with a friction strip or towel. Soak the skin in aromatic bathwater for a while before cleaning with friction.

Body wrap

A body wrap is the simplest and most effective way of decongesting the skin of the back and shoulders, especially if massage is not possible. Half-fill a basin with comfortably hot water and add 6 drops in total of juniper berry, lavender or rosemary. Stir the water to ensure that oils are fully dispersed and dip in a cotton towel big enough to cover the area. Wring out the excess water and spread the towel on the back and shoulders, ask somebody to put a sheet of plastic over the towel so that the heat of the towel is conserved. Relax for a while. You can use this treatment in a sitting or lying position. This draws impurities out of the body in a simple, relaxed way.

Aromatic back pack

An aromatic back pack is sort of messy but very helpful to refine the skin of the upper back, especially between the shoulders where sebum can clog pores and spots can accumulate.

The oils effective for an aromatic pack are mandarin, lemon, grapefruit, lavender, tea-tree, juniper berry and geranium.

Take 100 g of green clay

Add sufficient water to make a fine paste

Then add 5–6 drops of chosen essential oils

Mix together and apply. Leave the pack in place for half an hour, then shower it off. It is preferable and easier to dispose of dry clay instead of washing it down through the bathroom drain. The ultimate result of the back pack is tingling clean and clear skin.

Massaging the back and shoulders

A back massage with aromatic oil blends will mainly consist of effleurage and kneading of the areas of tension. A truly effective back massage will require around 20 minutes. The following massage blends can be used:

Relaxing blend
3 drops of sandalwood
3 drops of lavender
2 drops of geranium
15 ml of chosen carrier oil

Invigorating blend
3 drops rosemary
2 drops grapefruit
3 drops lemongrass
15 ml of chosen carrier oil.

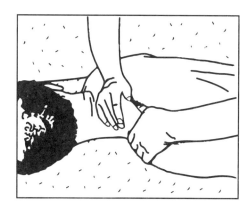
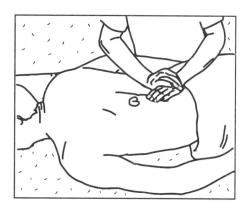

After the back massage, it is advisable to massage the points on the chest just above and below the clavicle towards the axillary nodes, as this is where the lymph drains into the bloodstream. Nature really is incredible: the main lymph drains are positioned on the front of the body where they can be reached easily. These points can be massaged at any time of the day. If you do not have access to massage, just apply the aromatic oil blend to the shoulder and neck where tension is stored and stiffness is often registered, then massage it down towards the axillary nodes.

Massaging, stroking and pressing different points around the neck, shoulders and upper back not only helps you to feel better, it helps relieve frozen shoulders to function more effectively in the long term.

TUMMY, WAIST AND ABDOMEN

The problems: Excess fat, fatty liver, wrinkles, tension stored in the solar plexus.

The causes: Fat deposits, toxic wastes, anxiety and stress.

The solutions: Aromatic bath, skin brushing, massage.

TUMMY AND WAIST

The tummy is often the first place we notice an increase in weight or girth. When skirts no longer fit and trousers will not zip up, we know that we have amassed excess fat. But why does fat accumulate so easily around the waist?

One reason may be that there are very few lymph nodes on the front of the torso. From the navel upwards, the lymph vessels take fluids and drain them to the axillary nodes under the arms, and from the navel downwards, the lymph drains to the inguinal nodes in the groin. Our inguinal nodes get blocked not only because of a sedentary lifestyle; emotional blockages also play a major role. Emotional blockages result in sacral (swadhisthan) chakra blockage, which causes energy congestion in the area and also blocks the lymph nodes. According to tantra, our sacral chakra controls the flow of fluids in the body including lymph. Lymph node blockages also affect the lower back, causing occasional pain in the lower back.

Because there are no lymph nodes actually at the waist, it is easy for cells to become crammed full of fat. By encouraging the flow of lymph to the nodes, which will filter and break down the fat deposits, we can help control the size of our waists.

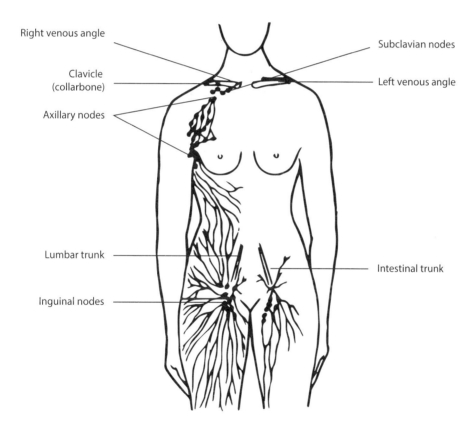

Aromatic baths

Bathe with oils such as juniper, lemongrass or fennel seed, which aid in the dispersal of unwanted fats and fluids. This helps to tone and firm the tummy, as fresh blood brings with it nutrients to feed the skin. Lymphatic movement is also stimulated, allowing fats to be broken down and carried away from the site, eventually to be expelled from the body. Many fats are recycled by the body simply because the liver is not able to cope with large quantities.

Release of emotional stress is of great importance when we are endeavouring to get rid of unwanted layers of fat. Stress affects people in different ways, and for some people too much stress can interfere with the efficient metabolism of the body, allowing a build-up of fatty deposits. As mentioned earlier, emotional stress causes blockage of the inguinal nodes. Mental stress also makes the solar plexus tight with bottled up stress, affecting diet and sleep. It is useful to add anti-stress oils to the bath, such as geranium, lavender and rose.

Skin brushing

Skin brushing of the abdomen is very effective because the concentration of the adipose fat makes it difficult for essential oils to penetrate. Skin brushing stimulates the movement of the fat and lymph, and encourages the drainage of unwanted toxins as well as the increased absorption of essential oils. If you intend to massage the tummy and waist later, skin brush the whole of the abdomen – the abdomen is the area from the diaphragm to the floor of the pelvis – as it will prepare the skin for the essential oil blends.

Take a brush and stroke from the navel downwards to the pubic area, brushing the skin across the inguinal nodes at the top of the legs. Then brush from the navel upwards to the diaphragm and, skirting around the breasts, sweep up to the axillary nodes at the armpit.

Massaging the tummy and waist

Massage of the tummy and waist can help to eliminate toxins, break up fatty deposits and encourage their dispersal, toning up the skin and underlying muscles so that wrinkles are reduced. The best way to massage the tummy is to start massaging the groin area (the inguinal nodes), as to move the stubborn fat it's important to unblock the lymph nodes first. Then massage the belly and push everything down towards the groin area.

If the flesh hurts when pinched between the thumb and fingers, this could indicate that the tissues are home to stagnant wastes, so choose the fat-burning blend. Choose the detox blend if you are prone to occasional water retention and the unwanted inches around your waist contain not only fatty tissue but also excess fluid.

Fat-burning blend	**Detox blend**
5 drops of lemongrass	5 drops of juniper berry oil
5 drops of grapefruit oil	5 drops grapefruit oil
5 drops of lemon oil	5 drops orange oil
5 drops of cypress oil	5 drops fennel seed oil

Add to 2 tablespoons (30 ml) of your chosen carrier oil (including at least 25% jojoba oil and 10% avocado oil).

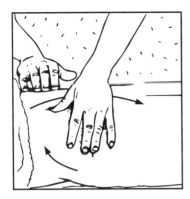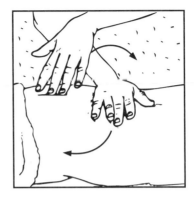

Wringing of the abdomen

Cling film wrap

The tummy and waist have so many fat cells clustered together that it is more difficult for essential oils to penetrate here. A cling-film wrap will aid the penetration of essential oils as well as encourage the elimination of water by causing the skin to sweat.

Firstly massage the waist with a blend of essential oils, such as the fat-burner blend or detox blend, then wrap a sizeable length of cling-film around the waist and tummy. A cling film wrap can be left in place for one or two hours, but for best results leave overnight, perhaps prior to a special occasion, when you want to squeeze into a figure-hugging item of clothing. If left on overnight, the essential oils will be unable to evaporate and will be forced into the skin. The skin will also sweat because of the close proximity of the plastic. After use, the cling-film should be cut and discarded. This is not a permanent way to banish fat from the tummy and waist but ideal for an instant tone-up and is a technique used in many beauty salons.

THE SOLAR PLEXUS

The solar plexus is sited halfway between the navel and the end of the diaphragm, and is a very sensitive area. If we are under stress or have experienced something traumatic (even watching the news on television) we may find that the area of the solar plexus is sore to touch. You may also find that just under the surface of the skin, this part of your abdomen feels tight and hard, as though the muscles have become 'knotted up'. This is precisely what has happened, but tension in the solar plexus can be very easily massaged away.

Solar plexus (self-massage)

Apply a little of the massage oil specified in the lemongrass and juniper mixes, above. Add 8 drops of lavender oil and 6 drops of geranium oil to the area between the navel and the sternum. Lie on the bed and rest your hand above the solar plexus and just breathe into the abdomen to the count of five, hold for the count of five, then exhale while counting to ten. Be aware of the tension under your hand.

Continue in this manner until the solar plexus has lost its tenderness, but at the most for 5–10 minutes. Finally, apply a little more massage blend and gently rub the abdomen, sweeping your hands in a clockwise circle. Rest for a few minutes, or make this the last thing you do before going to sleep, to ensure a restful night.

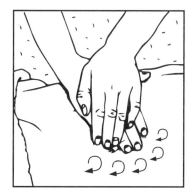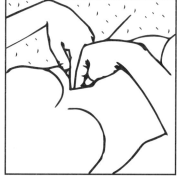

Massaging the solar plexus

THIGHS AND BUTTOCKS

The problems: *Thighs*: cellulite; dull, lifeless skin; excess fat (poor metabolism). *Buttocks*: Dull lifeless skin; pimples; buttock 'droop'; fat, cellulite and stretch marks.

The causes: Lymphatic congestion; stagnation – poor circulation; lack of exercise; poor metabolism and imbalanced nutrition.

The solutions: Aromatic bathing; skin brushing; friction massage; moisturising and nourishing massage.

CELLULITE

Cellulite is the term used to describe the pitted appearance of the skin. 'Orange peel effect' is an accurate description of the problem, and in France it is known as *peau d'orange*. Cellulite affects almost 60 per cent of women at some stage of the lives. Cellulite is not fat but the toxins embedded in the fat tissue. When the lymphatic system gets sluggish and not able to expel toxins, the body intelligence takes over and sends these toxins into the extremities so that they do not interfere with the normal functioning of the body and affect the vital organs. So it seems that buttocks and upper arms are the rubbish dump of the body.

Cellulite is most often found on the outside of the thighs, which can give our legs the appearance of wearing 'jodhpurs'. The sense of touch can detect the presence of cellulite, as the skin can be uneven and tender to the touch and if squeezed, very painful.

The good news is that cellulite is a condition which is not permanent and can easily be reversed with aromatic oil massage. Even though cellulite rarely responds to dieting and does not always respond to exercise, it does respond, fairly rapidly, to massage with specific essential oils, when rubbed towards the groin area to the inguinal nodes. This not only helps clear the cellulite also helps clear lymphatic congestion.

Cellulite is not a true disease in the sense of an irreversible pathological change, but a visual warning that the body is not functioning properly and those less-than-beautiful buttocks are trying to tell you that fat cells are accumulating on buttocks and upper arms.

Essential oils have the ability to decongest tissues and help the body to eliminate toxins, and often when the correct oil is chosen, both the internal problem and the skin condition is improved, as many skin problems have aromatic solutions. Essence of juniper berry and lavender are very powerful antiseptics but at the same time act gently on the skin; you can use these for baths and massage. Cellulite is a sign of congestion, visible on the skin, but the organs of elimination are affected. A juniper blend is used for massage of the affected areas. This has a draining effect and stimulates the flow of lymph.

In order to create an optimum situation for eliminating toxins, fats and excess water from the thighs and buttocks, the thighs must be skin brushed thoroughly, taking care also to brush the pubic area – the area of the body where the inguinal nodes are to be found. Stimulation of this area, followed by friction massage with specific essential and fatty oils, is a most effective way to banish cellulite from the thighs.

Cellulite blend
- 5 drops of juniper berry oil
- 5 drops of rosemary oil
- 5 drops of grapefruit oil
- 5 drops of cypress oil
- 5 drops of fennel seed oil

Add to 2 tablespoons (30 ml) of your chosen carrier oil (having at least 25% jojoba oil and 10% avocado oil).

OBESITY

Obesity is the result of eating more calories than the body can burn up through daily activity so instead of being used as fuel for energy, the fat cells become full and we become bulkier. The saying 'you are what you eat' is unfortunately very true.

Sitting for long periods every day and sedentary work are major factors in the loss of muscle tone in the buttocks. Toxins and fats are squashed by the weight of the body pressing down on a relatively small area of the buttocks. The upper thighs also suffer from prolonged periods of sitting, especially the back of the thighs, where the circulation can be seriously impaired by pressure from the edge of a chair.

For obesity and lack of muscle tone, stubborn areas of fat will respond to physical massage, especially when used with essential oils that have a stimulating effect on the metabolism, such as grapefruit oil for the gall bladder, juniper for the kidneys, and lemon/orange for the liver. A fat-burning blend used in the regular massage of the thighs and buttocks has a very toning and slimming effect.

Daily massage therapy for obesity
- 5 drops juniper berry oil
- 5 drops lemongrass oil
- 5 drops grapefruit oil
- 5 drops lemon oil
- 5 drops rosemary oil

Add to 2 tablespoons (30 ml) of your chosen carrier oil (having at least 15% jojoba oil and 10% avocado oil).

STRETCH MARKS

If the living skin is considerably overstretched by rapid weight gain or loss, ruptures can occur in the structure of the corium, which become visible as pale, silvery stripes, so-called 'distension striae', commonly known as stretch marks. Stretch marks often accompany cellulite or excess fat in the thighs.

The dermis is a dense network of collagen fibres, intermingled with elastic fibres that allow the skin to stretch and return to normal. The cells that originate in the basal layer of the epidermis undergo a step-by-step transformation leading to the migration of cells from the bottom layer to the surface, a process which takes about 30 days. This means that by applying essential and fatty oils in generous amounts, over a period of time, we will be able to influence the new growth of cells that will replace the ruptured skin tissue, and the stretch marks will eventually disappear. However it is a slow and time-consuming process.

With all problems of the thighs, massage with the fat-burning blend (see page 251) can be very successful. When massaging, focus should be unblocking the inguinal nodes. Once you've tackled the cellulite and reduced the excess fat, massage with the following blend:

Stretch mark blend for thighs

- 5 drops of cedarwood
- 5 drops of geranium
- 5 drops of lavender
- 5 drops of rosemary
- 5 drops of vetiver

Add to 50 ml of your chosen base oil (with 10% calendula added to help the stretch marks recede and become less visible).

Aromatic bathing

The morning is an ideal time of day to tackle cellulite and excess fat on the thighs and buttocks. Skin brushing and the choice of essential oils are all fairly stimulating.

Add to the bath those essential oils that are refreshing and uplifting. The zest of oranges or mandarin is a natural choice to revitalise and set the mood for positive action. To this you could add a few drops of geranium, if your emotions need a 'lift'.

Massaging the thighs

Using either the fat-burning blend or the detox blend (see page **253**), apply a little at a time, to one thigh, noting how it seeps into the skin. Beginning just above the knee, work the oil into the skin in small patches, and continue to build up further areas of oiled skin until the entire thigh has been covered. Reposition your leg as necessary, to gain access to every part of the thigh. Using fingertip pressure, stroke the fingers up the leg, not too forcefully and not too gently either. You will be able to feel areas of discomfort and nodules of fat under the skin. Continue to apply more of the massage oil blend, working it into any 'problem areas'. Be sensitive to your body, spending more time massaging sore spots, before sweeping the palm of the hand up the thigh to the top of the leg, and ending the massage over the pubic area and inguinal nodes. This area may feel sensitive and tender to the touch. The fat-burning blend is preferred as we want to 'spring clean' the connective tissue and allow the powerful lemongrass oil in the blend to 'burn up' the toxins that have accumulated over the years. The citrus oils in the blend will cleanse, detoxify and help the body's lymphatic system to drain more easily.

MASSAGING THE BUTTOCKS

If your buttocks have lost their youthful curves, and the buttock cheeks no longer have firm definition but droop and merge ingloriously into the back of the thighs, then this area deserves attention. It is possible to rejuvenate the buttocks and bring back a firm contour, but only with consistent effort: by working on this area with the massage oil blends, and exercising.

Using either the fat-burning or the detox blends from page **251** as preferred, massage the oil into one buttock, adding more oil as it is absorbed by the skin. The best way to self-massage the buttocks is to be semi-reclining. Lie on top of your bed, on your side, with the buttock to be worked on uppermost and the leg bent.

Use your fingertips to massage and work the oil blend into the entire skin surface, paying particular attention to the area where buttock meets thigh. Use firm circular strokes here and focus on any portion of skin that feels knotty or lumpy. Even after only a few sessions of massage to this area, a difference can be seen in the shape and definition of the cheeks, and if the buttocks are massaged regularly, it is possible to regain a youthful contour.

KNEES, ANKLES AND FEET

The problems: Fat knees, puffy knees, wrinkly knees; puffy ankles, hidden ankles; corns and callouses; cracked feet; tired feet; nail bed infections.

The causes: Poor metabolism, hormonal imbalances, excess fat, lymphatic congestion, dehydrated skin, age, ill-fitting shoes, neglect.

The solutions: Aromatic bathing, skin brushing, lymphatic massage, footbath.

KNEES

Even a woman with the most shapely legs and gorgeous figure can feel let down by her knees, especially when her legs are bare. There are lymph nodes under the knees called popliteal nodes, and congestion of these lymph nodes coupled with the congestion of the inguinal nodes is the major cause of puffy or fat knees. Fortunately essential oils work on a deeper level on the skin of the knees, just as they can on the face or any other part of the body. The most common problems are fat knees, puffy-looking knees or wrinkly knees. In all knee problems, aromatic bathing and skin brushing are the first step, followed by massage with a well-chosen blend of essential and fatty oils.

Aromatic bathing and skin brushing

The emphasis is on skin brushing. Take your nailbrush and brush up the leg from ankles to knees, using medium pressure. Then brush across and around the knee as well as underneath the knee, where the popliteal lymph nodes lie. Next, bend the knee, and with firmer pressure, brush the top of the knee from all sides, and take the brushstrokes about a third of the way up the thigh. Finish the skin brushing by stroking the bristles along the pubic area to the inguinal nodes.

The skin may look pink and feel hot, which is a good sign because blood is being brought to the surface of the skin. This has two effects: it brings nutrients to the skin surface and it prepares the skin for the essential oil massage.

Massaging the knees

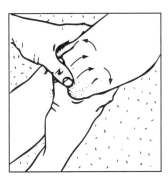 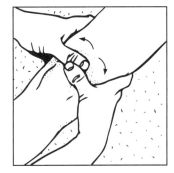

Fat knees: First, feel the underside of your knees: feel the congestion of your popliteal nodes at the underside of the knees. You may find the underside of one or both the knees swollen: that's the sign of congestion of lymph nodes. A massage with the fat-burning blend (see page 251) is excellent for this, as it decongests and detoxifies the area. Simply massage the underside of the knees in a circular motion and pump to move the lymph through to the thighs and to the inguinal nodes. It's a good idea to massage the inguinal nodes in circular motions to unblock them before massaging the knees.

Puffy knees: Puffy knees will definitely have congested lymph nodes under the knees. A massage with the detox blend is helpful for anyone who experiences fluid retention around the knees. This is a common but easily resolved problem, so take heart.

Wrinkly knees: Age and dry skin produce knees that look a little wrinkled. Like wrinkles on the face, a firm massage with a vetiver oil blend containing 7 drops of vetiver, 3 drops of geranium, 3 drops of cedarwood and 3 drops of lavender in 2 tablespoons of your chosen base oil (containing avocado and jojoba oils along with olive or grapeseed oil) can restore a youthful, firm texture to these trouble spots.

ANKLES AND FEET

Being even further from the torso than the knees, the ankles and feet can easily accumulate fluids (especially premenstrual), fats and toxins. Dry brushing and a foot soak with essential oils followed by scrubbing, and then massage with aroma oils is very helpful.

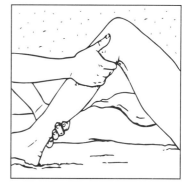

Massaging the ankle to knee.

Footbaths and skin brushing

You can use any essential oil blend for a footbath. In summer, peppermint with rosemary is a cooling and uplifting combination. In the winter, oil of myrtle with black pepper is comforting and warming. Anyone who suffers from foot odour can use cypress, juniper or frankincense, since these oils have natural deodorant properties. It is also recommended to add a tablespoon (15 ml) of Epsom salts to the footbath.

With a nailbrush, brush the top of the foot from the toes to the ankle, paying particular attention to the area around the inside and outside of the ankle bone. Most of the lymph from the foot drains to the popliteal nodes, but some lymph vessels go directly to the inguinal nodes. Therefore, stimulate both areas with the nailbrush.

Puffy ankles

Make a foot soak with 3 drops each of juniper berry, cypress and pine needle oil, then follow it with gentle massage. The detox blend (page 253) is wonderfully effective, as the juniper oil in the blend is a good diuretic and helps drain fluid from this area. Long hours of standing or after a party or other occasion when larger than normal quantities of alcohol have been consumed, the ankles become a little puffy – this is the body's way of saying it is having difficulty in coping with the alcohol. Drinking extra glasses of water is a valuable aid to your body's elimination system, as is a massage with a diuretic essential oil blend.

Hidden ankles

Either excess fat or water retention is the cause of hidden ankles. Massage with either the fat-burning or detox blend (see page 251) to help uncover ankle bones you'd forgotten you had.

Massaging the ankles and feet

Apply the chosen oils to the top and sides of one foot and ankle. With firm fingertip pressure, stroke from the toes to the ankle, and then draw your fingers around the ankle. Massage in a circular motion around the ankles. Continue these movements for several minutes. Apply the maximum pressure you find bearable; some of us have very sensitive feet and ankles, but the massage should have a degree of firmness. If the feet and ankles are massaged on a regular basis, they become less tender to the touch as toxins and fluids are removed. Finish the massage by smoothing the skin up to the knees, so that the lymph is encouraged to drain. As some lymph vessels drain directly into the inguinal nodes, be sure to massage this area as well. Many women experience swelling and tenderness of the flesh just below the ankle bone immediately prior to menstruation, and gentle massage of this area will help the body to release tissue fluids.

Tired feet

Lots of tension is stored in the feet, not to mention the trauma of teetering around on high heels, or simply standing on and using the relatively tiny feet to support the body's weight. They need a treat from time to time. Nothing is lovelier than an aromatic foot soak. Place your feet in a few inches of warm water to which Epsom salts and a few drops of essential oil have been added, such as lavender, geranium, ylang-ylang, juniper berry or bergamot.

After a 10-minute soak, use a pumice stone to smooth away dry skin from the heels and toes. Cover one knee with a towel and put your other foot up for a massage. Clench your fist and, starting at the base of the toes, draw your knuckles along the length of the foot to the heel. Cover the whole foot with knuckle caresses, which stimulate many foot reflex points and release tension. Change the towel to the opposite knee and do your other foot. Dry the feet with the towel and apply a little jojoba oil. You should feel as though you are walking on air!

Corns and callouses

Corns and callouses are the result of ill-fitting footwear causing friction at the pressure zones at the sole of the foot, resulting in hardening of skin. Direct application of tea-tree or in combination with oregano and calendula is useful. You can also use salicylic acid (or aspirin powder) to make a paste and apply to the corn, or use a corn plaster onto which 1 or 2 drops of tea-tree oil have been dripped.

Cracked feet

Excessive dryness and metabolic deficiency causes the cracking of the skin especially around heals, due to body weight. Soaking, moisturising and nourishing the feet is helpful in correcting this condition. Beeswax, avocado oil, jojoba oil, almond oil, water and essential oils are useful ingredients to make an emollient and protective foot cream:

- 15 g of beeswax (finely chopped)
- 1 tablespoon (15 ml) of jojoba oil
- 1 tablespoon (15 ml) of avocado oil
- 2 tablespoons (30 ml) of almond oil

Place in a bowl in a double boiler at medium heat and allow to melt, stirring occasionally. After it has melted, remove the bowl. Let it cool a bit then add a little hot water (at the same temperature), whisk to make an emulsion, add essential oils and store in a jar. Keep in a cool place away from light and heat. Alternatively use 1 teaspoon (5 ml) each of almond oil, jojoba and avocado oil as a base to which you can add 3 drops of vetiver, 3 drops of patchouli and 3 drops of lavender. Apply thoroughly after a foot soak.

Nail bed infections

Nail bed infections are usually fungal in nature, due to wearing synthetic socks for much of the time, or to moisture. The best treatment is to use neat tea-tree oil, apply 1–2 drops on the affected nails two to three times daily. Tea-tree oil can also be used in a foot soak. Follow with a foot massage then apply additional tea-tree oil to the affected nails.

Athlete's foot

This is a contagious fungal infection characterised by red, flaky skin and itching. Athlete's foot occurs between the toes, sometimes affecting the toenails.

Make a blend using 1 teaspoon (5 ml) of almond oil and 1 drop each of lavender, oregano, myrrh and tea-tree. Apply at least 3 times a day.

Tea-tree may also be applied neat (or diluted in a gel) – check sensitisation first by patch test.

UPPER ARMS, ELBOWS AND NECK

The problems: Saggy upper arms, cellulite, obesity, wrinkled elbows, rough or dead skin on elbows, dehydrated skin, stored-up tension in neck, lines on neck.

The causes: Loss of muscle tone, toxins, poor metabolism, age, pressure of leaning (elbows), emotional and mental stress, and poor circulation.

The solutions: Bathing, skin brushing, massage, astringent mask, moisturising.

Aromatic baths

Bathing in aromatic water is beneficial for all problems relating to the upper arms, elbows and neck. Only a few drops of essential oil to a full tub of water are needed to create a therapeutic bath that will cleanse the skin, relax tense muscles and open up the pores of the skin in readiness to receive massage oils. Many essential oils are excellent for the skin but especially recommended for their therapeutic properties and their fragrance: try rosemary, orange, geranium, juniper berry, ginger and lavender.

Skin brushing and massage

Skin brushing and massage release toxins from the body by the gentle stimulation of the skin's surface, and when incorporated into an aromatic bathing ritual, transforms the process of taking a bath into a health and beauty treatment.

Take a nailbrush and brush from wrist to elbow, gently at first, as many times as it takes to cover the entire forearm. Then repeat using firmer pressure. Gently brush the folds of the elbow, where the cubital nodes are housed. These lymph glands are the first line of defence in detoxifying our hands, nails and forearms, and can become swollen and painful and also lead to painful fingers. Now sweep from the bend of the elbow up to the top of the arm, if necessary lifting up your arm so that you can brush the underside axillary nodes. Continue the gentle brushing and sweep the armpit, so that the axillary nodes are encouraged to work efficiently in carrying away the waste material dislodged by massage. Finally, sweep across the top of your shoulder, from the base round to finish where the arm meets the body. Relax in the aromatic water for five minutes or so. Repeat on the other arm. You can massage the wrists to elbow joints and then up to the axillary lymph nodes.

Massaging the neck is helpful: focus on the occipital nodes and massage gently, then bring it down through the shoulders to the underarms. The neck can also be skin brushed in the bath, with the brush stroking downwards from under the skin of the chin to the base of the neck. Work your way around the neck until all the skin, even the back of the neck, has been brushed. Next, sweep the brush from the back of the neck round to the front, finishing where the two ends of the clavicle meet. Using slightly firmer strokes, brush from the shoulder across the front of the chest, under the clavicle, and end at the top of the sternum. Repeat on the other side of the body.

UPPER ARMS

Cellulite on upper arms: Cellulite on the upper arms is the body's 'overflow' tip, where it dumps toxins that it cannot deal with in other ways. The fat-burning or detox blends (see page 251) will remove toxins from the connective tissues, deep cleanse and disinfect the dermis and bring a fresh supply of blood to the surface of skin, helping the circulatory system to carry away unwanted debris.

Excess fat on upper arms: Too much fat on the upper arms probably occurs in tandem with too much fat on other parts of the body. The fat-burning blend is most suitable for massage, in this case. Allow your fingertips to detect the condition of the underlying skin; feel the lumps under the surface and encourage them to go away. If there are tiny spots or hard crystal-like deposits under the skin, encourage their removal and elimination by massage.

Saggy upper arms: We say that something is 'saggy' when it has lost its tone and succumbed to the forces of gravity. Saggy upper arms are usually seen on women who have lost not only weight but also muscle tone, either from age or from crash dieting, leaving the skin to hang in folds. Some improvement in the appearance of the upper arms can be achieved with massage of the skin with the detox blend. However, it will only be possible to effect a very gradual change in the condition and appearance of the skin, and best results will be achieved if a little light exercise is also incorporated, along with a testosterone supplement.

Dry skin: Dry, wrinkly skin is the easiest of the upper arm problems to rectify, as dry skin denotes a lack of oils in the skin. Skin cells are constantly renewing themselves. As the old, dead cells are removed from the surface of our bodies, new cells are already being pushed upwards, towards the surface. By feeding the skin with pure oils, both essential and fatty, we can feed the deeper layers where the cells are formed, giving them the ideal conditions for birth and growth. Essential oils of vetiver, sandalwood and cedarwood combined with base oils of almond, avocado, wheatgerm and jojoba oil will give the skin all the nourishment it requires, while the vetiver in the blend will encourage the cells to absorb and retain moisture, making them and more youthful.

Massaging the upper arms

Whether your upper arm problem is cellulite, excess fat, saggy loose skin or rough dry skin, the massage technique is the same. Massage of the upper arms, following an aromatic bath and skin brushing, is the most effective way to get essential oils into the skin.

With your choice of either the fat-burning or detox massage blend (see page 251), apply the oil to the upper arm, from the elbow to the shoulder to the underarm to the axillary nodes. Rest the left wrist and hand across the top of the head – this will enable you to massage the underarm more easily. Using only your fingertips, smooth and stroke the skin from the elbow to the armpit with short and repetitive strokes, like sweeping leaves along the ground. Be sensitive to your body and feel for any little fatty bumps, crystals or pimples under the surface, and massage these areas thoroughly. Apply more oil blend whenever necessary. Dropping your arm down by your side, massage the outer edge from elbow to shoulder, smoothing away the lumps and bumps.

Now turn the arm so that the palm is facing upwards and massage the biceps. Again using fingertip massage, work the oil blend into the skin from elbow to shoulder. Finish by massaging the entire armpit area and help your axillary lymph nodes to carry out their important function.

Do not shave, wax or use depilatory cream on the underarms immediately before or after massage of the upper arms and underarm area.

ELBOWS

It is sometimes said that a person's true age can be determined by looking at their elbow, because the elbows cannot be cosmetically enhanced and cared for in the way that the face can.

The flesh covering the elbow is, by necessity, fairly loose-fitting, as elbows have to bend. It can therefore easily lose elasticity and become wrinkled. Whatever problem we experience with the condition of our elbows and upper arms, a regular massage with an essential oil blend in the morning and evening will help. However, it may take some time to have a noticeable improvement both in the appearance and feel of the elbows.

Puffy fat elbows: Puffy and fat elbows are unlikely to be found in isolation, and will be part of an overall excess of adipose tissue in the body. The true solution for puffiness lies in eating healthily and increasing the body's metabolism, but a useful aromatic adjunct is to massage the elbows with the fat-burning blend of oils (see page **251**). It will help the lymph to take away fluids and proteins and return them to the circulatory system where they may be further broken down and eliminated from the body.

Hard, dry and wrinkled elbows: As with dry upper arms, the problem of dry elbows is a lack of natural oil, which in mature skins is added by a breakdown in connective tissue and inability to retain moisture. The blend of vetiver in jojoba and avocado oil is a wonderful combination for massaging dry, wrinkled elbows, since vetiver can help the skin cells to attract and hold water more easily. Sandalwood is another useful oil for massaging into dry skin.

Massaging the elbows
The main problems are puffy or fat elbows and hard, dry and wrinkled skin. Although seemingly

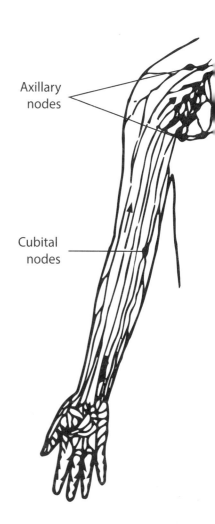

Axillary nodes

Cubital nodes

different, the cause is fairly constant buildup of toxins, fluids or fats due to inadequate lymph drainage and lack of physical care. Massage of the elbows with the detox blend (page 253) and stimulation of the cubital lymph nodes (in the fold of the elbow) will help to bring about a more healthful, youthful appearance. Whatever the individual problem, the massage technique is the same: fingertip massage, using the chosen aromatic blend, and lots of it.

Pour a little blended oil into a small massage bowl. Sit on the edge of your bed or chair with the left arm crossing in front of your body and the left hand resting on your right forearm, and smooth the oil into the skin around the right elbow. Using the fingertips, massage the flesh around the bony part of the elbow, feeling how much or how little flesh is covering the bone. While smoothing in the oil, feel for any little bumps or hard spots under the surface of the skin. These are not supposed to be there and denote the presence of pockets of toxins, excess proteins, knotted fibres and crystal deposits. Now, with your fingertips, stroke and rub the skin on and around the elbow, giving extra attention to rough or lumpy areas. Continue the fingertip massage for 10–15 minutes. Then, stretching out your right arm, massage the inner elbow where the cubital lymph nodes are housed. These nodes are responsible for the health of our forearms, hands and nails, filtering away toxins and producing lymphocytes. Using the flat of your hand, stroke the flesh upwards from below the elbow to the top of the arm and finally spend a minute or so massaging the nodes at the top of the arm, lifting up the right arm and rubbing the nodes at the junction of the arm and the torso. Now change hands and massage the left arm in the same way.

NECK

Whether long and sleek or short and thick, our neck supports our head, enables us to see around corners, and is a place of adornment. Like the elbows, the flesh covering the neck has to be fairly loose in order that we may have 180-degree flexibility to the left and right. The skin of the neck is a dense network of collagen fibres, intermingled with elastic fibres, which enable the skin to stretch and then return to normal. Small enough to be encircled by our two hands, the neck houses an incredible collection of bones, veins, arteries, nerves, glands, lymph nodes and ducts, as well as the gullet and windpipe. The muscles of the neck have to support the weight of the head (around 4 kg) which is why too much strain or tension in the neck produces a headache. Emotional or mental stress aggravate the condition.

Stretching the neck from time to time is beneficial to the muscles and the blood flow, and especially important if our job causes us to sit for many hours a day with our heads facing in one direction, such as in front of a computer or TV screen. Massaging the neck is also important for several reasons: to release tension from the muscles; to encourage the free flow of lymph, and the efficient drainage of waste products from the head, face and the neck itself; to allow good blood circulation; and to prevent any impingement of nerves. Looking after the neck is much more than just a cosmetic routine to enhance our physical beauty; it is a sensible way to keep the face, head and whole of the body in a good state of health.

Lines and loose skin: The neck should ideally be cleansed and moisturised every night as part of the daily care plan for the face. The skin on the neck, like the skin of the face, is subject to contact with polluted air and the elements, and will need to be thoroughly cleansed every day. After cleansing, apply 3 drops of vetiver, 3 drops of lavender and 3 drops of rosemary in 1 tablespoon of olive and jojoba blend, then using large, firm sweeps, massage into the sides of the neck. With long hair pinned up, massage the back of the neck, at the occipital area, from the hairline down to the shoulders, and rub away at any sore spots your fingers may discover. There are many lymph nodes in the neck that draw toxins from the face and head.

Massaging the neck

Ideally the front of the neck should be cleansed and massaged every day at the same time as your face. In this way the skin stands the very best chance of retaining its elasticity and staying free from lines. However, the back of the neck at the occipital nodes will only need to be massaged periodically, such as when you have a headache, or when you want your neck and shoulders to look as good as your face.

By massaging the back of the neck at the occipital nodes with a massage

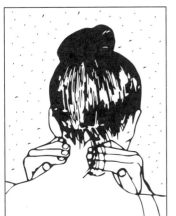

oil blend, we can release a lot of tension, relax sore and tight muscles, and encourage the dispersion of toxins and static energy, so easily accumulated by hours of desk work, driving, worrying over problems, or even just by sleeping in the wrong position at night.

You can even use neat lavender oil for the purpose, as lavender releases the stiffness of the muscles. Alternatively prepare a blend using essential oils of lavender, myrtle, rosemary, juniper berry and geranium in a base oil of olive, grapeseed and avocado.

Apply a little of this blend to the fingertips and place your hands on the back of your neck so that your fingers meet on the vertebral column. Now draw the fingers down, round and up so that the neck is being covered in large circles, and continue to do this for as long as you feel comfortable. Next, stretch hands even further down the back of the neck and starting at the spine and applying firm pressure, down your fingers, round the bottom of your neck, until they reach the right angle between neck and shoulder.

Repeat this move several times as it is a very effective way of removing tension and allows energy to flow to the head. Next, place fingertips at the base of the neck and slide them up the back, with fingers on either side of the spine. When your fingers reach the hairline, apply stronger pressure and hold for a count of five. Allow your fingers to press and soothe all sore spots along the occipital bone (where the skull joins the neck) and continue outwards until your hands reach your ears. Then, taking the back of the neck between fingers and thumb, squeeze gently, allowing your fingers and thumb to slide across the skin and meet at the spinal column. Finish the massage by stroking the fingers from the top to the bottom of the neck and applying firm pressure to the lymph nodes below the clavicle.

HAND AND NAIL CARE

The problems: Dry skin, dehydrated skin, fat or puffy hands, brittle nails, ridged nails.

The causes: Lack of moisture, insufficient sebum production, environment, diet.

The solutions: Aromatic hand bath, nail soaks, moisturising, massage barrier cream.

HANDS

Hands and face are the two areas of our body most often exposed to the elements. Even if we are blessed with a youthful-looking face, our hands can instantly reveal our true age. While we protect our facial skin with moisturisers and make-up, our hands are often neglected and become damaged. There is only a thin layer of flesh over the bones of the hand and the back of our hands can age more quickly than the skin of the face. Even if we are blessed with a youthful-looking face, our hands can instantly reveal our true age.

There are two ways to improve your hands:

1. A barrier cream applied regularly throughout the day.

2. A nightly moisturising routine with rejuvenating oils and aromatic waters.

Daytime barrier cream

A barrier cream has two functions. Firstly, to provide an invisible film or barrier against the environment, the weather, central heating or air conditioning and water in all its usages (such as washing up, washing our hair and handling the laundry). Secondly, to soften and moisturise dry skin and feed it with nourishing fatty oils and essential oils.

Beeswax, jojoba oil, almond oil, water and essential oils make an inexpensive emollient and protective hand cream:

- 15 g of beeswax (finely chopped)
- 1 tablespoon (15 ml) of jojoba oil
- 3 tablespoons (45 ml) of almond oil

Place in a bowl in a double boiler at medium heat, allowing to melt, stirring occasionally.

After it has melted, remove the bowl. Let it cool slightly, then add a little hot water (at the same temperature) and whisk to make an emulsion. Stir in your chosen essential oils (see below) and store in a jar in a cool place away from light and heat.

This is simple to make and contains no preservatives, so it is preferable to make a small batch every 3 to 4 weeks, rather than a large one infrequently.

There is a huge range of essential oils that could be chosen for their fragrance, as well as their ability to soften and protect the skin, including vetiver and lavender or geranium with sandalwood. Warm, earthy aromas, such as vetiver, patchouli and sandalwood, make a pleasing bouquet when blended.

Night-time rejuvenating hand massage

Massage the hands before going to bed using a vetiver oil blend. Hold your left hand with your right, and with the right thumb massage the back of the hand using small circular movements, working between the carpal bones. Take one finger of your left hand between the fingers and thumb of your right hand and massage the entire length of the finger. Rub your palms together and smooth the oil into the entire hand and wrist. Repeat on the other hand. When dry, apply a little more vetiver oil blend. After massaging the hands, spend a few minutes massaging the lymph nodes situated in the elbow area.

Hand bath

Hands that are dry, rough or damaged can be healed and softened by the use of an aromatic hand bath. Any of the essential oils that are beneficial for dry skin may be used, such as sandalwood, rose, vetiver, lavender, geranium or patchouli. Alternatively, use a combination of rosewater with a little glycerine.

To prepare a hand bath, you will need a bowl that is large enough to place both your hands in comfortably for 10–15 minutes (a casserole dish may prove to be the correct size). Essential oils differ in their ability to disperse in water and if using one of the viscous oils – sandalwood, vetiver or patchouli – it will first be necessary to mix them with a thinner oil such as lavender, geranium or palmarosa. Place essential oils in the bowl, add warm water and allow your hands to soak for 10–15 minutes.

Choose either of the following combinations:

- 1 drop vetiver
- 1 drop sandalwood
- 2 drops geranium

Or

- 2 drops rose or geranium
- 2 drops lavender
- 2 drops frankincense

Pat hands dry with a clean towel and apply a liberal amount of jojoba or argan nut oil. Massage it into the hands, as if washing your hands with the oil, until they have absorbed as much oil as possible. Rub excess oil onto any other area of dry skin, such as the elbows or knees, or alternatively blot the excess with a tissue.

THE NAILS

The nail is composed of keratin, as is the skin; it is a horny plate of the epidermis. It consists of cornified scales overlapping like roof tiles. The nail bed is the living part of the nail and consists of connective tissue channels that carry blood vessels along the nail's length, from the half-moon to the fingertip. It is the flow of blood beneath the surface of the nail that gives the pink or red tinge. The nail projecting from the fingertip is completely dead, which enables us to cut and file our nails without experiencing pain.

Nothing much can be done to increase the strength of the nail once it has grown beyond the fingertip, but much can be done to grow healthy nails in the nail bed. When nails are dry and brittle and split easily, it is simply because they are not receiving sufficient 'food' in order for them to grow. A vitamin A supplement will also help to improve the condition of nails. The aromatic way to bring nutrients to the nail bed is to use sweet almond oil or natural vitamin E oil.

Massage oil for nails
A simple but effective massage oil for nails can be prepared in minutes:
    1 tablespoon (15 ml) of sweet almond oil
    1 teaspoon (5 ml) of wheatgerm oil
    1 teaspoon (5 ml) of jojoba oil
    4 drops of lavender oil
    3 drops of geranium oil
    2 drops of sandalwood oil.

Dip the fingertips into the mixture so that some oil goes under the nail. Next, massage the oil into the nail wall, half-moon and up to the first joint of the finger. When the mixture has begun to be absorbed, put your fingertips together so that your hands form a sphere, and gently press the nails of the right hand under the nails of the left hand. Hold for a few seconds. Then press the nails of the left hand under the nails of the right hand.

Aromatic nail soak

An alternative to using the massage oil for the nails is to soak the fingertips in a pot of warm water containing:

- 2 drops of lavender oil
- 2 drops of geranium oil
- 3 drops of wheatgerm or vitamin E oil (optional)

Both lavender and geranium are tissue stimulants, and promote the growth of new skin – one of the reasons why they are used to heal burns. By soaking the fingertips in this aromatic liquid (especially if vitamin E is included), a highly nutritious meal is provided for our nails. Allow nails to soak for 10–20 minutes, depending on how starved your nails are. Rinse your hands in clear water after soaking, pat dry, and massage in a little jojoba oil or aromatic barrier cream.

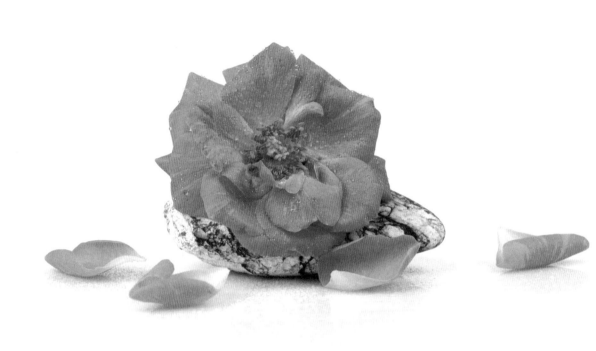

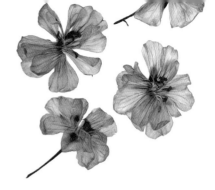

PURELY FOR PLEASURE

Experimenting with the aromatic potential of essential oils can be fun. The oils can be blended in infinite combinations to produce individual perfumes, room fragrances, bath essences and more. Producing a personal fragrance is also a creative and educational experience.

CREATING YOUR OWN PERFUME

Indian attars were initially designed as therapeutic perfumes, using essential oils depending on the season. Certain essential oils like jasmine, sandalwood and rose can be worn straight or diluted in jojoba oil as a personal perfume or you can blend a few oils together to create your signature perfume.

The different depths of fragrance in a blend are called 'notes' and each scent takes on a particular character according to the balance of base, middle and top notes from which it has been made. Top notes are those light oils that evaporate quickly, like lemon, melissa, neroli, bergamot or grapefruit. The middle notes provide the heart of a blend and include oils like lavender, geranium or rosewood. The heavier base notes linger for hours, and act as the fixative for the other lighter oils. Traditional base notes are viscous oils like sandalwood, patchouli, vetiver, myrrh and benzoin. A well-balanced fragrance should contain elements from each group.

APHRODISIACS

Certain oils have a reputation for increasing sexual desire, including cedarwood, ylang ylang, jasmine, neroli, patchouli, rose, sandalwood, clove and frankincense.

- Use 5–10 drops of a combination of jasmine, ylang ylang and neroli in the bath to create a romantic atmosphere.
- You can also create a combination of these oils to vaporise in the bedroom to create a sensual mood, or use in your wardrobe to scent linen or clothes (it will also protect them).
- The spice oils, which include black pepper, cardamom, clove, nutmeg and ginger, are also reputed to have aphrodisiac properties. However, because they have strong natural chemicals that may cause skin sensitisation, they should be used only in moderation: 3 drops in the bath or 1–2 drops added to other blends.

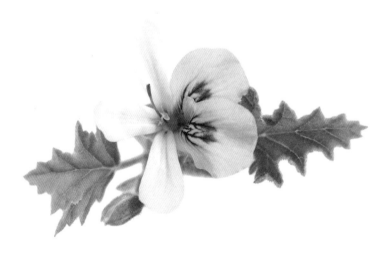

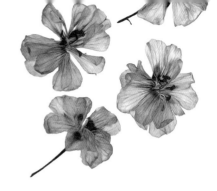

PART IV

THE TREATMENT OF COMMON AILMENTS

Aromatherapy, the art and science of healing and rejuvenation, can be used by all therapists, medical or non-medical, as a complementary therapy for the prevention and treatment of common and chronic ailments. As mentioned in earlier chapters, aromatherapy oils and products boost the immune level, help eliminate toxins at a fundamental level and aid healing, as well as providing specific therapeutic effects according to the properties of the oil used. These common conditions respond well to aromatherapy:

First aid: Cuts, burns, bumps, insect bites, sprains, cramps etc.

Beauty/facial care: Helps with ageing, wrinkling, dark under-eye circles, pigmentation and scars/marks. **Aids with** dandruff, hairloss and greying.

Chakra healing/balancing: Essential oils are the subtle life force of the plant so a potent tool for chakra healing and balancing.

Infections: Essential oils are reputed to be anti-infectious, antibacterial, antiviral and antifungal, therefore effective in **post-operative care.**

Skin disorders: Including eczema, psoriasis, **fungal infections, non-healing ulcers, bedsores,** boils, acne, herpes, corns, warts, scars, sunburn and nail bed infections.

Muscular problems: Including aches, pains, sprains, cramps, rheumatism, arthritis and bursitis (tennis elbow).

Circulatory problems: Including blood pressure related (high/low), palpitations, hypertension, varicose veins and piles/fistula.

Respiratory conditions: Including asthma, bronchitis, sinusitis, common cold, and respiratory tract or lung infections.

Psychosomatic conditions: Stress, anxiety, depression, hypertension, headaches, migraines, insomnia and fatigue.

Gynaecological conditions: Candida (thrush), leucorrhoea, cystitis, pruritus, oedema, **PMS** and menstrual (period-related) problems.

Other problems: Eg mouth ulcers, tooth and gums infections, laryngitis, pharingitis and even digestive problems.

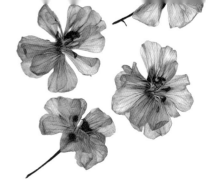

FIRST AID AND MUSCULAR PROBLEMS

BRUISES AND BUMPS

- Lavender oil is one of the best for bumps, bruises, cramps and sprains. For quick pain relief, and to stop the swelling, apply neat lavender.
- Minor bruises and bumps can be treated using a cold compress (such as a wet flannel or lint wrapped round an ice cube) with 3 drops of either lavender, marjoram or geranium.
- If there is inflammation, 2 drops of German or Roman chamomile should be applied, along with 5 drops of lavender, in 1 teaspoon (5 ml) of non-greasy cream or gel.

BURNS (MINOR) AND SUNBURN

- For minor household burns or scalds, apply ice-cold water immediately for 10 minutes, then a couple of drops of neat lavender. Renew 3 times daily.
- Large areas of redness from sunburn can be soothed by adding 5–10 drops of German or Roman chamomile to a lukewarm bath and soaking for 10 minutes. More severe patches or blisters should be treated with a few drops of neat lavender oil.

- A good after-sun treatment for dry, parched or red skin is to blend 2 drops each of lavender, geranium and German or Roman chamomile with 1 tablespoon (15 ml) of almond oil or aloe gel. Massage in well after sunbathing.

CUTS, SORES AND SCARS

- Essential oils are very useful for minor first aid since they can reduce the possibility of infection, encourage the skin to heal and help prevent scarring.
- Always clean a cut or sore carefully with a little cooled boiled water to which has been added 2 drops of any of the following antiseptic oils: lavender, tea-tree, juniper or geranium.
- For small cuts or grazes, apply 1–2 drops of neat lavender as needed. For larger injuries, add a few drops of lavender and tea-tree to a plaster or gauze to cover the wound. Renew the dressing 3 times daily.
- For infected cuts or splinters, apply 3 drops of tea-tree and 1 drop of German chamomile diluted in 1 teaspoon (5 ml) of gel to the affected area 3 times daily, especially if there is inflammation.
- If the wound is bleeding, dab it with gauze soaked in a bowl of cold water to which has been added 2 drops each of lavender, tea-tree and cyprus.
- If the cut or sore is weepy, a drop of oil of myrrh, benzoin or patchouli may be applied to the dressing or used to bathe the wound, in combination with 2 drops each of lavender and tea-tree, diluted in warm water.
- For bedsores and non-healing ulcers, a combination of lavender, tea-tree and German chamomile with calendula is very effective.
- If a scar is slow to heal, make an ointment using 3 drops in total of either German chamomile, lavender or frankincense (or a

combination of these) in 1 teaspoon of wheatgerm oil mixed with a little calendula or rosehip oil. This should be applied regularly until the skin is healthy again.

INSECT BITES AND REPELLENTS

- When it comes to treating bites or stings, the simplest, most effective remedy is neat lavender, applied immediately to the sting and then re-applied at least 3 times a day. This works for mosquitoes, gnats, bees, wasps and ticks (as well as nettle rash). For ticks, apply a drop of neat tea-tree to make them lose their grip, then remove.
- If there is a rash, swelling or inflammation, 1 drop of German or Roman chamomile and 2 drops of lavender should be added to 1 teaspoon (5 ml) of non-greasy cream or gel and applied.
- To keep insects out of the house, vaporise a combination of any three of the following oils: citronella, lemongrass, thyme, peppermint, lavender, basil, eucalyptus, geranium or Atlas cedarwood. You can also use them in plant sprays or apply to hanging ribbons.
- An excellent blend can also be made by mixing 2 drops each of thyme, lavender and peppermint with 8 drops of lemongrass. This can be used as an airborne deterrent: blend in an oil burner, vaporiser or plant sprayer. You can also add 6 drops to 1 tablespoon of carrier oil or cream, to be applied directly to the skin.
- A simple method of keeping insects at bay, especially mosquitoes, is to rub a few drops of neat lavender onto exposed areas of the skin or clothing (it does not stain).
- Oils that keep moths away from linen include lavender, patchouli, camphor, Atlas cedarwood and basil.

MUSCULAR ACHES, PAINS AND SPRAINS

- Muscular pain as a result of overexertion responds well to local massage. To ease aches and pains, use 3 drops each of lavender, rosemary, wintergreen and eucalyptus in 1 tablespoon olive oil, then rub into the affected areas well.

- Soaking in a hot bath is an easy and effective way of bringing instant relief. To aid relaxation and ease pain, add 5–10 drops of lavender, eucalyptus, marjoram, clary sage and basil to the water. Adding Epsom salts to the water will help to relax the tired muscles.

- To relieve muscle spasms, apply neat lavender as first aid or in combination with marjoram and eucalyptus in olive oil. Alternatively, add these oils to a hot compress.

- To help prepare the muscles for action and increase muscle tone, use 3 drops each of rosemary and juniper with 2 drops of black pepper in 1 tablespoon (15 ml) of carrier oil for local massage; or add 5–10 drops of rosemary, grapefruit or juniper to the bath.

- To treat a sprain, apply lavender oil directly or prepare a cold compress to which has been added a few drops of either lavender or German chamomile (or both). Apply to the injury and repeat as often as possible to reduce the swelling. Do not massage. Wrap in a bandage and rest the joint as much as possible.

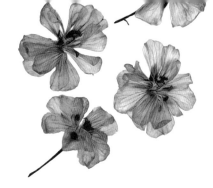

PAIN RELIEF WITH ESSENTIAL OILS

Pain is generally an acute and unpleasant sensation arising from bodily injury or disease. Concepts of pain and pain mechanisms are highly controversial and for that reason all classifications of pain remainarbitrary. The bony framework of the skeleton is covered by voluntary muscles that we can contract or relax at will. In contrast, the involuntary muscles of the heart and digestive system are outside our immediate control. Pain may be experienced in either. For treatment of any pain, the following three things should be ascertained first:

Position of the pain: Locate the area of greatest severity as accurately as possible, often suggestive of the disease.

Character or severity of the pain: Ascertain how it interferes with sleep, pleasure or work.

Nature of the pain: Translate as far as possible the symptoms into scientific terms. Diseases that cause little pain in the beginning may end fatally.

For practical purposes, there are two principal types of pain: superficial and deep. Pain is sharply localised in superficial structures like the muscles and joints, or diffusively localised in deeper structures like the heart and digestive system. Usually relief from pain is achieved by removal of the stimulus or neutralisation of the effects of the stimulus, and when these are not feasible, by dulling or obliterating the sensation of pain.

Essential oils administered for pain relief work on the muscular system by neutralising or removing the stimulus, besides helping to remove the underlying cause of the pain. If the cause of the pain is disease or illness, only proper diagnosis and treatment can help. Pain also forces the patient to rest the part that is diseased. Nothing can undermine the importance of rest. Indeed, rest is the first principle in the treatment of all diseases. Essential oils may be used in addition to relax muscles, relieve pain, and cleanse and detoxify the system, since essential oils work on our body at the fundamental level by improving circulation, increasing the body's regeneration rate and eliminating toxins. All essential oils, by their nature, are antiseptic, antibacterial, antiviral and disinfectant. Some also have special therapeutic properties including anti-inflammatory, warming, stimulating, diuretic, analgesic or muscle-relaxant. One of the most renowned oils for all kinds of pain, especially rheumatic pain, is essential oil of wintergreen, mostly used as methyl salicylate (active ingredient of the oil) in pain balms and liniments. However, when we use a combination of aromatherapy oils such as wintergreen, eucalyptus, rosemary, marjoram, clove, lavender or thyme in a suitable carrier oil, the results are much more efficient.

CRAMPS

Temporary muscular spasms during or after physical exertion are not uncommon, but a more long-term problem is the type of cramp that occurs in the evening or at night, affecting mainly the calf muscles and feet, thought to be due to poor circulation or possibly calcium and potassium deficiency. Application of neat lavender helps this condition; other useful oils to relieve this type of cramp are sweet marjoram, basil, cajuput, eucalyptus, rosemary and chamomile. The essential oils can be mixed in a suitable base oil and rubbed well into the area. Those who are prone to this type of muscular cramp can make and keep this mix ready and handy. As a preventive measure, the oil blend can be applied every night initially, later the frequency reduced to every second night then twice a week; if cramps return, increase the frequency of application.

SPRAINS

A sprain may occur when ligaments are torn or stretched by a sudden jerky movement. The affected joint becomes swollen and painful. Sprains respond well to aromatherapy treatments: neat lavender can be used on the affected area as a first aid. Seek medical attention if there is a possibility of a broken or splintered bone.

To treat a sprain, prepare a cold compress to which essential oils of sweet marjoram, rosemary, lavender and German chamomile are added and apply to the affected area. You can also prepare a mix of these oils in a suitable base oil for gentle application to the affected part. Never massage a sprained joint. Repeat the compress as often as possible to reduce swelling. Wrap in a bandage and rest the affected part as much as possible.

RHEUMATISM, ARTHRITIS AND BURSITIS

Rheumatism is a general word for pain and inflammation affecting the joints and surrounding muscles, and includes arthritis and bursitis. Arthritis is a term used to describe inflammation of the joints. There are two main types: rheumatoid arthritis is a chronic inflammation of the connective tissue around joints, which causes pain, swelling and stiffness, and is often accompanied by weight loss and tiredness. It seems to affect women more than men and, unlike osteoarthritis, usually attacks pairs of joints. Conflict on an inner or emotional level often contributes to the development of this disease, as does a poor diet, which can lead to a build-up of toxins in the body, with uric acid being deposited as crystals in the joint spaces. Climate is also an important consideration, and humidity aggravates the condition. In severe cases, the joints can become crippled and deformed. Ingestion of

1 teaspoon (5 ml) of evening primrose oil per day helps the condition.

Osteoarthritis is a progressive wearing away of the cartilage, which results in severe pain and reduced mobility. The connective tissue thickens and fluid may fill the joint, causing swelling. Aromatherapy can help to relax muscles and relieve pain, but it cannot renew worn cartilage nor can it always help to relieve pain in the bone. However, oral consumption of gum acacia (babool gum) helps repair the cartilage. Another effective treatment includes 1 teaspoon (5 ml) of evening primrose oil taken orally every day, along with calcium supplements. Evening primrose not only helps calcium absorption but also regulates the body's physiology.

Bursitis is one of the most common rheumatic conditions, usually affecting the shoulders, elbows (tennis elbow) and knees (housemaid's knee). A combination of 3 drops each of lavender, eucalyplus, wintergreen and rosemary oils in 2 tablespoons (30 ml) of olive oil can be rubbed in the affected area and massaged to the nearest lymph nodes.

Essential oils for rheumatic conditions

One of the renowned essential oils for rheumatic conditions and inflammation is oil of wintergreen, which can be combined with eucalyptus and rosemary and used in conjunction with other oils like German chamomile. In the case of swelling, juniper berry, eucalyptus, rosemary, and cypress are also useful. The warming properties of black pepper, sweet marjoram and ginger help to relax muscles and relieve mild pain.

Prepare a calming, anti-inflammatory and detoxifying massage mix using 5 drops each of juniper berry, eucalyptus, lavender, pine needle and German chamomile oil in 3 tablespoons (45 ml) of olive oil. This mix can be applied with gentle pressure but avoid massage of painful or inflamed joints. Warm baths can also help to relax muscles and relieve pain. Just sprinkle a couple of drops each of lavender, rosemary and eucalyptus in the bathwater. In a hot compress, using a couple of drops of black pepper, lavender, or marjoram, or a combination of these, helps to ease local pain.

A good antirheumatic oil for general application is 2 drops each of lavender, rosemary, pine needle, wintergreen, juniper berry and eucalyptus, prepared in 1 tablespoon (15 ml) of a suitable carrier oil.

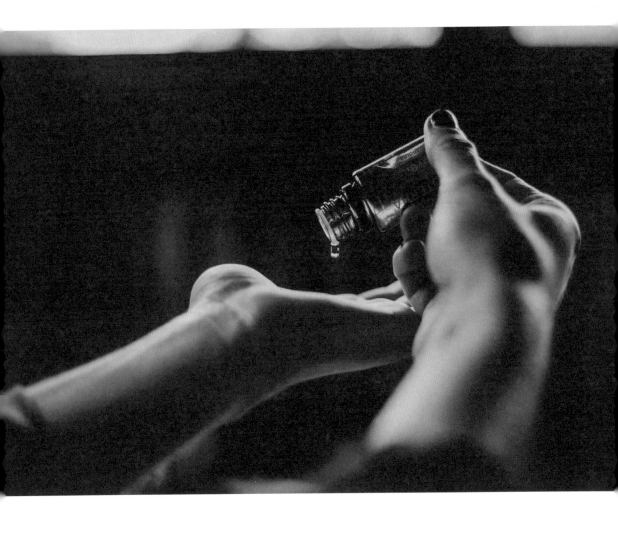

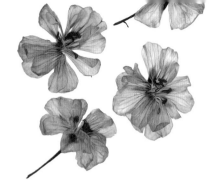

INFECTIOUS AND RESPIRATORY ILLNESS

ASTHMA AND HAYFEVER

Asthma, characterised by attacks of wheezing and shortness of breath, is very often an allergy-induced disorder, starting in childhood and frequently going hand-in-hand with bronchitis, hayfever and other allergic reactions, such as eczema. An attack can be triggered by an infection like a cold or by allergens such as pollen or dust, but it is also largely related to overexertion and stress, especially in those of a nervous disposition.

Hayfever is due to an allergic reaction to pollen or other irritants, and since some essential oils can induce allergic reactions, extreme care must be taken in the choice of oils. The following combinations can help to alleviate the problem, but because asthma and hayfever affect people in different ways, the treatment is often a case of trial and error.

- The most useful oil for hayfever and asthma is peppermint, as it is antispasmodic (soothing), expectorant and helps to clear the head. Use regularly in the bath (3 drops only) and also use in a vaporiser or on the pillow.
- Oral ingestion of evening primrose oil helps boost the immune system, regulates the body's physiological functions and controls allergic reactions.

- Other soothing oils, such as clary sage, frankincense, lavender, mandarin, neroli and rosemary can all help to ease nervous tension or anxiety: add 5–10 drops to bathwater or vaporise.
- Regular massage, especially on the chest and back, using a relaxing, soothing blend can help prevent tension and anxiety building up. A recommended mixture is 2 drops each of frankincense, thyme, rosemary and lavender in 1 tablespoon (15 ml) of carrier oil.
- During an attack of asthma and hayfever, sufferers can put the following oils on a tissue to inhale: 3 drops in total of peppermint, frankincense, cajeput or rosemary (or a combination of these).
- For everyday use, add a few drops of frankincense, geranium, lavender, peppermint and eucalyptus to a vaporiser to create a relaxing atmosphere in the home.

COMMON COLDS AND SINUSITIS

The two most useful oils for stimulating the immune system and fighting the cold virus are eucalyptus and tea-tree. Combine them with lemon (the limonene in lemon oil boosts the antiviral properties of eucalyptus oil) and frankincense. At the first sign of a cold appearing, use these oils in a vaporiser or apply a few drops to the pillow or a tissue for inhalation throughout the day and night.

- For shivers, headaches and aching muscles, take a warm bath with 3–5 drops each of lavender, basil, ginger and marjoram. This will also encourage restful sleep.
- Eucalyptus, rosemary, lemon, basil, peppermint and bergamot help to reduce temperature and fight infection. A few drops of these oils can be used in a vaporiser or added to a dish of steaming water placed in the sickroom.
- The best way to combat congestion, sinusitis and catarrh is to use steam inhalations. Add a few drops of rosemary, peppermint

or eucalyptus to a bowl of hot water and inhale deeply for 3–10 minutes, keeping eyes closed. In addition, use the above oils in a vaporiser or add a few drops to a tissue for inhalation throughout the day.

- To further clear the head of stuffiness and help fight viral infection add 3 drops each of rosemary, peppermint and lavender or cajuput with pine needle to a steaming bath.

- For a sore throat, add 3 drops in total of clary sage, sandalwood, tea-tree or geranium (or a combination of these) to a glass of warm boiled water, with a little fresh lemon juice (an excellent antiseptic). Mix well and gargle. (Not to be used by children under five).

COUGHS AND BRONCHITIS

Coughs can be dry and irritating or they can be accompanied by mucus discharge, especially in association with a cold or with bronchitis.

Bronchitis indicates an inflammation of the bronchial tubes, accompanied by coughing and an overproduction of mucus. Acute bronchitis usually starts with a cold or sore throat, which then develops into a fever that lasts a few days. Chronic bronchitis is a long-term condition, without fever, which is aggravated by smoking, a damp climate, air pollution and poor nutrition (especially too many dairy products).

- When there is fever present, eucalyptus, tea-tree, lemongrass, thyme, peppermint and bergamot help to reduce temperature and fight infection. A few drops of these oils can be used in a vaporiser or added to a dish of steaming water placed on a radiator in the sickroom.

- The best way to combat excess mucus, congestion and catarrh is to use steam inhalations. Add a few drops of rosemary, holy basil, peppermint or eucalyptus (or a combination of these) to a bowl of hot water and inhale deeply for 3–10 minutes, keeping the eyes closed. In addition, add a few drops to a tissue for inhalation throughout the day.

- There are many essential oils with balsamic properties that are soothing and help to loosen mucus (for dry or irritating coughs). The most effective are rosemary, myrtle, eucalyptus, myrrh, frankincense, holy basil, sandalwood and pine needle. A few drops of any of these oils can be used. Alternatively, for a dry cough, simply add 3 drops each of pine needle, holy basil, eucalyplus and frankincense in a vaporiser or to bathwater.

- A local back and chest massage oil, which is effective against bronchitis, coughs and catarrh, can be made by blending 2 drops each of eucalyptus, juniper berry, holy basil, frankincense and ginger with 1 tablespoon (15 ml) of olive oil.

- A useful oil for nightly coughs in children and adults is myrtle, since it helps to fight infection but is not too stimulating, which might otherwise prevent sleep. Use a few drops on the pillow or on nightclothes or in a vaporiser.

FEVER AND INFECTION

Although essential oils can help provide relief during an infectious illness, as well as reduce its duration and prevent it from spreading, in cases of high fever, severe infection or an acute childhood illness, the following home treatments should not be used as a substitute for professional help.

- The most useful oils for stimulating the immune system and fighting viruses of all kinds, including the flu, are eucalyptus combined with lemon oil and tea-tree. Use these oils in a vaporiser in the sickroom or put a few drops on the pillow or on a tissue for use throughout the day and night.

- For shivers, headaches and aching muscles, take a warm bath with 4 drops each of lavender, ginger, holy basil and marjoram. This will also encourage restful sleep. Roman chamomile is helpful in overcoming anxiety or insomnia.

- When there is fever present, eucalyptus, tea-tree, lemon, thyme, peppermint and bergamot help to reduce temperature and fight infection. A few drops of these oils can be used in a vaporiser or added to a dish of steaming water placed in the sickroom.

- For a sore throat, add 2 drops in total of clary sage, holy basil, sandalwood, tea-tree or geranium (and a little fresh lemon juice) to a glass of warm boiled water, mix well and gargle. (Not to be used by children under five).

MOUTH, TOOTH AND GUM INFECTIONS

A traditional remedy for toothache is to put 1 drop of clove oil on a cotton bud and apply to the tooth. (Do not swallow. Not safe for children, as they may swallow.)

- Disease of the gums (gingivitis) is a common cause of tooth loss, and care of the gums is vital to health. A good mouth rinse to prevent bleeding or swollen gums is 3 drops in total of cypress, clove, tea-tree, lemon, sandalwood or thyme (or a combination of any three of these) in a cup of warm boiled water together with a pinch of sea salt. If the infection is severe, a few drops of neat tea-tree oil should be massaged on the affected area.

- To treat mouth ulcers, dry the affected area and dab twice daily with tea-tree or myrrh. You can use the same oils along with cypress in warm water for a gargle.

- For swelling and pain resulting from infected gums or wisdom teeth, mix 3 drops in total of clove, tea-tree and cypress in 1 teaspoon (5 ml) of carrier oil, and massage into the cheeks. A cold compress also helps ease pain.

- A good remedy for bad breath or halitosis is to use the following mixture regularly: 100 ml of inexpensive vodka, 10 drops each of lemon and peppermint or spearmint, and 5 drops each of cypress, tea-tree and juniper berry. To use, mix 2 or 3 teaspoons (10–15 ml) in half a cup of warm water, and rinse the mouth out twice daily.

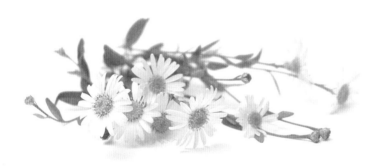

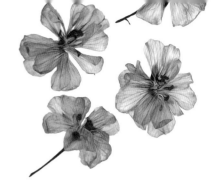

STRESS-RELATED CONDITIONS

With the present-day emphasis on materialism and the achievement of external goals, it is important to keep in touch with ourselves on an inner level. Allowing space for ourselves is something that many of us find difficult, whether because of work or family pressures. Stress is the modern-day disease, and one we all suffer from at some time or another. When we are stressed our energy level dips and our immune system gets compromised, and we become less resistant to all kinds of illness that affect the body, the emotions and the mind. A lot of modern illnesses are called 'psychosomatic' in origin – in a sense starting at a mental level and finally showing in the physical body.

The use of aromatics can help to lift anxiety and bring about a change in our state of mind. This is one of the most traditional uses of essential oils, and the reason they have played an important role in both religious and spiritual rituals for thousands of years. Engaging in the ritual of a candlelit aromatic bath, burning essences to create a relaxed atmosphere in a room, or using essential oils for massage or to aid meditation, are all ways of slowing down the mind and becoming more attuned to the moment. It is also important, of course, to try to deal with the causes of stress directly and if necessary seek professional help.

Because of the emotional elements at play in stress-related conditions, the choice of essential oils depends largely on the causes of the problem, as well as the temperament of each individual and how they respond under pressure. The following aromatic recipes may provide a few ideas.

DEPRESSION AND ANXIETY

Depression can take many forms, and it is important to try to understand the causes and deal with them directly. Essential oils can help alleviate the symptoms, but since this is primarily an emotional complaint, the method of treatment is very much an individual matter.

- If the depression is associated with lethargy and lack of energy, oils such as sweet/holy basil, bergamot, geranium, rosemary, neroli, jasmine and rose can be uplifting and energising. Jasmine oil has been clinically trialled as an antidepressant; it works well in a blend with neroli and ylang ylang. These can be used in the bath, in a vaporiser, or as perfumes. Practising massage either on oneself or with a friend can be of great benefit, combining both the comforting effect of touch and the remedial effect of the oils.
- If the depression is associated with restlessness and anxiety, then the more sedating and soothing oils, such as chamomile, clary sage, lavender, Atlas cedarwood, marjoram, vetiver, ylang ylang and sandalwood, can help encourage a relaxed state of mind. Aromatic baths, massage, scenting the home and using essential oils as perfumes are all ways of bringing enjoyment and pleasure both to the individual and to those around them. Jasmine, melissa and lemongrass, along with all citrus oils, have been found to be good antidepressants. The oils that are traditionally used as incenses, such as benzoin, Atlas cedarwood, patchouli, frankincense, juniper and sandalwood, can help bring about a calm state of mind, used either as perfumes or in a vaporiser. Since there are so many oils to choose from when it comes to helping depression, one of the best

ways of deciding is simply to select the scent that appeals and gives a lift to the emotions in that moment.

DIGESTIVE UPSETS

Digestive upsets are often the result of stored anxieties. They respond well to the external application of essential oils, but this is often enhanced by the use of herbal remedies, such as peppermint, chamomile or fennel tea.

- Stomach-ache of nervous origin can be helped by gentle massage to the abdomen, especially in the area of the solar plexus, in a clockwise direction using 9 drops in total of marjoram, rosemary, lavender, fennel or thyme (or a combination of these) in 1 tablespoon (15 ml) of carrier oil. Neroli or black pepper are also soothing in cases of nerves or emotional upsets. Use in the bath, as vaporised oil or in a massage combination.

- For indigestion with wind, use 3 drops each of fennel, juniper berry and spearmint in 1 tablespoon (15 ml) of carrier oil for abdominal massage (clockwise) as indicated above.

- To help ease constipation, use 3 drops each of marjoram, thyme and fennel seed in 1 tablespoon (15 ml) of carrier oil for abdominal massage (clockwise).

- If there is diarrhea or a viral infection is suspected, use 3 drops each of tea-tree, juniper, oregano and thyme in 1 tablespoon (15 ml) of carrier oil for massage (anticlockwise) on the abdomen.

- The other spice oils are also very beneficial to help relieve pain and promote digestion, used in minute amounts in massage oils or baths. They include black pepper, carrot seed, clove, cardamom, cinnamon, coriander and ginger.

FATIGUE, POOR CIRCULATION AND LOW BLOOD PRESSURE (HYPOTENSION)

Fatigue can be caused by exhaustion and stress, or can be related to feelings of lethargy due to a slow metabolic rate. Poor circulation and low blood pressure often occur together, and in both cases stimulating essences are advised. Attention to diet and exercise is also very beneficial, especially for those with a sedentary lifestyle.

- Rosemary is the most useful oil for this condition, being stimulating and tonic. Use 5 drops each of rosemary, black pepper and holy basil and in the bath.
- A vigorous massage using 5 drops of rosemary, 2 drops of lemongrass or melissa and 2 drops of black pepper in 1 tablespoon carrier oil also helps to stimulate the system.
- Exhaustion and fatigue of a more emotional nature can be helped by mentally reviving and uplifting oils such as jasmine, holy basil, bergamot, neroli, melissa or geranium, used in vaporisers or as perfumes.
- Excessive fatigue can be counteracted with refreshing and uplifting bath oils, which may be used in the morning or before going out in the evening after a heavy day. Recommended bath blends are 3–5 drops each of rosemary, geranium, mandarin and holy basil; rosemary, melissa and lemongrass or petitgrain; or a combination of geranium, neroli and holy basil.

HEADACHES AND MIGRAINE

For tension headaches, apply neat lavender to the temples or to the back of the neck. To ease strain and tension, massage the shoulders and neck using 1 teaspoon (5 ml) of carrier oil with 3 drops each of lavender, holy basil and marjoram.

- For congested headaches due to blocked sinuses, use a few drops of peppermint with eucalyptus on a tissue to inhale throughout the day. These oils can also be used in a vaporiser or added to a bowl of steaming water as an inhalation.

- Migraine is the result of an imbalanced solar plexus chakra, caused by diet, mental stress, heated liver and sometimes due to hormonal imbalances, as is the case in menstrual cycle-related migraines in women. A cold compress placed on the temples using 1 drop of lavender and peppermint, can help to ease discomfort during an attack. As a preventive measure, soothing and relaxing oils such as lavender, Roman chamomile, basil and marjoram should be used on the temples and solar plexus area. It also helps to change the breathing nostril to control the migraine.

HIGH BLOOD PRESSURE (HYPERTENSION)

Although aromatherapy treatments have been found to reduce blood pressure significantly, it is also vital to review issues such as diet, exercise and general lifestyle. Certain breathing exercises help regulate blood pressure, and important among those is alternate nostril breathing. In addition, garlic, either eaten raw or taken as pearls or tablets, has been found to help reduce cholesterol and control high blood pressure. Stimulants, such as tea, coffee and alcohol, should be reduced or eliminated. Evening primrose oil taken orally (1 teaspoon/5 ml daily) along with lecithin also helps to regularise blood pressure.

- Regular massage is particularly helpful for this condition and can dramatically reduce high blood pressure – an excellent blend for massage at home is 3 drops each of ylang ylang, lavender, clary sage and marjoram in 2 tablespoons (30 ml) of carrier oil. Massage this blend on the soles of the feet and around the chest to the underarm towards the axillary lymph nodes.

- The use of other relaxing and sedative oils such as bergamot, Roman chamomile, patchouli, vetiver or sandalwood is also effective. Use 5–10 drops of any of these oils (or a combination of them) in the bath, in a vaporiser or as a perfume.

NERVOUS TENSION AND INSOMNIA

For the workaholics, some good soothing bath combinations to use before retiring are 2–3 drops each of lavender, vetiver or sandalwood with Roman chamomile and patchouli. Other oils also very beneficial for relaxation are geranium, clary sage, ylang ylang, neroli and Atlas cedarwood.

- Emotional stress and nervous tension expresses itself in different ways. Some people cope by becoming overactive, some people become depressed, while others collapse. Some good basic bath combinations that are supportive and comforting are 3–5 drops each of bergamot, geranium and neroli (antidepressant), or sandalwood, lavender and geranium (soothing, relaxing), or jasmine, ylang ylang and geranium (uplifting and stimulating).
- A full body massage at the hands of a qualified aromatherapist can do much to alleviate stress, but massage can also be carried out in the home. A recommended blend for general tension/irritability is 3 drops each of lavender, geranium, ylang ylang, sandalwood and clary sage in 2 tablespoons (30 ml) of carrier oil.
- Tension is often held in the body, especially in the neck and shoulder areas. A good massage blend for easing muscular tension and general aches and pains is 3 drops of rosemary, marjoram, lavender or a combination of these in 1 tablespoon (15 ml) of a suitable base oil.
- The best oils for the insomnia that often accompanies stress are lavender, clary sage, marjoram, ylang ylang and patchouli. Use in the bath, or put a few drops on the pillow or in a vaporiser in the bedroom before retiring.

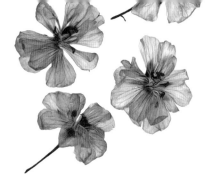

WOMEN'S HEALTH

CELLULITE

Although aromatherapy is very successful in helping to combat cellulite, this obviously needs to be supported by exercise, dietary measures and, if possible, professional lymphatic massage. Hormonal imbalance, as well as stress and too much tea, coffee and alcohol, which all increase toxicity levels, also contribute to this condition.

This stimulating, toxin-eliminating oil blend should be used on successive days: 3–4 drops each of rosemary, juniper, lemongrass, fennel seed and grapefruit added to 2 tablespoons (30 ml) of base oil and massaged into the thighs and buttocks up to the inguinal lymph nodes every day. This can also be applied to a loofah or massage glove and rubbed into the affected areas while bathing.

CYSTITIS AND PRURITUS (ITCHING)

Cystitis, which is an infection of the bladder, is characterised by a painful burning sensation while passing urine. Pruritus, or itching, is an irritating condition that often accompanies a mild vaginal infection. Take garlic pearls, drink plenty of water and keep tea, coffee, alcohol and spices to a minimum. Avoid tight-fitting clothes and nylon underwear.

- For cystitis, make up a solution (well shaken) using 5 drops each of tea-tree, palmarosa or geranium, sandalwood and bergamot in 500 ml of cooled boiled water. Using a piece of soaked cottonwool, swab the opening of the urethra frequently (if possible, each time after passing urine).
- In addition make up a massage oil, using 3 drops each of German chamomile, juniper berry, tea-tree, sandalwood and lavender, with I tablespoon (15 ml) of carrier oil. This blend should be massaged into the lower back and abdomen twice daily.
- To help combat cystitis and pruritus, it is beneficial to bathe frequently using bactericidal essential oils. Add 5–10 drops of a combination containing lavender, German chamomile, juniper, sandalwood and tea-tree to a warm bath, or add 2–3 drops to a bidet for localised washing.

MENSTRUAL PROBLEMS

Essential oils can help to combat menstrual disorders on a variety of levels because they are able to operate on the emotional and the physical areas simultaneously. One of the most useful oil for all kinds of menstrual problems is clary sage.

- For period pain, gently massage the lower abdomen and lower back with a blend containing 3 drops each of lavender, clary sage and marjoram in 1 tablespoon (15 ml) of base oil.
- Alternatively, add a few drops of clary sage and marjoram to a hot compress, and apply to the abdomen.
- The effects of premenstrual tension can be eased by taking regular aroma baths with oils that help to relieve tension. Add 5–10 drops of one of lavender, clary sage, neroli or rose to the bathwater. In chronic cases, 1 teaspoon (5 ml) of evening primrose oil, taken orally, for a period of 3 months, helps a lot.

- To help regulate heavy flow, make a massage oil blend using 3 drops each of cypress, geranium and clary sage, in 1 tablespoon (15 ml) of carrier oil and rub anticlockwise, on the lower abdomen. In addition, use 5–10 drops each of these oils in the bath.
- Diet, exercise and emotional factors should also be assessed.
- To normalise scanty menstruation, make a massage oil blend, using 3 drops each of clary sage, juniper berry and Roman chamomile in 1 tablespoon (15 ml) of carrier oil to rub clockwise on the lower abdomen. In addition you can use 5–10 drops each of these oils in the bath. Poor diet, anaemia and being rundown often accompany this problem so diet and other lifestyle factors should also be assessed.

OEDEMA (WATER RETENTION)

Although this is not an exclusively female complaint, oedema often occurs during the later stages of pregnancy. It may also be caused by being overweight or other factors such as food allergies, standing for long periods or hormonal imbalance. It most commonly occurs in the legs around the ankles and knees; but can also be found in the hands, stomach, or around the eyes.

- The most useful oils are juniper berry, fennel, cypress, geranium and rosemary. Add 9 drops of a combination of these to 1 tablespoon (15 ml) of carrier oil or cream and massage gently at the site of the swelling. Legs should be massaged with upward strokes.
- Alternatively, massage the soles of the feet with 2–3 drops each of juniper berry, cypress and lavender, in 1 tablespoon (15 ml) of carrier oil.
- For swollen ankles, submerge in a lukewarm footbath containing Epsom salts and a few drops of juniper berry, cypress, fennel, geranium or rosemary.

- Take warm baths containing 5–10 drops of the aforesaid oils in combination.
- Swelling and puffiness can also be relieved by applying a cold compress using 1 teaspoon witch-hazel lotion with 2 drops each of juniper and cypress to the affected area.

LEUCORRHOEA AND CANDIDA (THRUSH)

Leucorrhoea is an inflammation of the vagina caused by the proliferation of unwanted fungi, resulting in a thick white or yellow discharge.

Thrush is a form of fungal infection which affects warm, moist parts of the body, but most commonly occurs in the vagina, where symptoms include itching and a thick milky discharge.

Both conditions are aggravated by tight clothing, nylon underwear, harsh bubble baths and the use of antibiotics. Most cases of thrush and leucorrhoea respond well to the use of tea-tree oil.

- Add 5–10 drops of tea-tree to the bathwater daily or a few drops to a sitz bath for a localised wash. (Check sensitivity first.)
- Make a douche by mixing 10 drops of tea-tree with 500 ml of cooled boiled water and bathe the area using an enema pot, or soak a tampon in the above solution and insert into the vagina.
- Other oils of benefit that may be used in the bath include geranium, juniper, lavender, sandalwood and bergamot: add 5–10 drops to the bathwater.

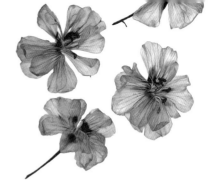

PREGNANCY AND CHILDBIRTH

PREPARING FOR MOTHERHOOD

More and more women are choosing to deliver their babies in as natural and as active a way as possible, without the use of drugs. There are now many books available on the subject, which cover issues such as nutrition, exercise or herbal remedies, all of which can help to make pregnancy and the birth easier and more enjoyable. Essential oils are being used increasingly by nurses and midwives in this context.

Using essential oils during pregnancy to help with childbirth can be very beneficial in a variety of ways, but there are some precautions to be taken, due to the sensitivity of the womb and the unborn foetus.

1. Use all essential oils at half the usual stated amount during pregnancy.
2. Oils that should be avoided altogether are basil, cinnamon, citronella, clary sage, clove, hyssop, juniper, marjoram, myrrh, Spanish sage, tarragon and thyme.
3. The oils that are best avoided during the first 4 months of pregnancy are cedarwood, fennel, peppermint and rosemary.

PREGNANCY

An excellent oil to help prevent stretch marks can be made by blending 2 drops each of lavender and palmarosa or geranium with 1 drop each of neroli and frankincense, added to 1 teaspoon (5 ml) of wheatgerm oil or rosehip seed oil, plus 1 tablespoon (15 ml) of olive oil – for light massage daily of the belly and breasts. This oil can also help to lighten existing stretch marks.

- In addition, wheatgerm oil can also be rubbed into the perineum to help prepare for the birth. Research has shown that massaging the perineum for 5–10 minutes daily in the last 6 weeks of pregnancy can help prevent tearing.
- Aromatic bathing offers great pleasure and relief, especially towards the end of pregnancy. Add 3–5 drops of any of the following oils to the bath: uplifting oils like bergamot, neroli, mandarin, geranium and jasmine or relaxing oils like sandalwood, rose, lavender, patchouli, ylang ylang and frankincense.
- Pamper yourself during pregnancy using the following essential oils as perfumes or as soothing air fresheners to overcome anxiety and encourage a relaxed attitude to the forthcoming birth: lavender to relax; Roman chamomile, vetiver or sandalwood to calm the mind; bergamot, neroli and mandarin to uplift; rose or jasmine to comfort.
- Gentle massage can be very enjoyable during pregnancy, and can help with a wide variety of problems, such as back pain. To soothe back pain and relax the body, lie on one side and ask a friend or partner to apply the following blend to the lower back: 3 drops each of lavender and Roman chamomile in 1 tablespoon (15 ml) of nourishing base oil.
- Oedema, fatigue, varicose veins, constipation and other digestive problems are also common during pregnancy (individual ailments

are covered elsewhere in Part IV). Always take care to avoid contraindicated oils, and use in low dilutions only.

LABOUR

- A traditional and useful massage oil to help prepare for the birth and strengthen the uterus muscles is a blend of 2 drops of jasmine or neroli with 1 drop of nutmeg in 1 teaspoon (5 ml) of nourishing base carrier oil. Rub the oil on to the lower abdomen each day for 2 weeks prior to the expected delivery.
- During the birth and when preparing to bring the baby home, the use of vaporised oils to scent the environment can create an uplifting, relaxed mood. They also prevent the spread of airborne bacteria. Use a few drops of lavender, frankincense, mandarin or bergamot in a vaporiser, or in a bowl of hot water.
- Pain relief during labour can be aided by firm massage to the lower back using the following blend: 3 drops of lavender and 2 drops each of geranium and rosemary in 1 tablespoon (15 ml) of carrier oil.

AFTER THE DELIVERY

- To help heal the perineum after the birth, add 2 drops of cypress and 3 drops of lavender to a sitz bath, and soak. Repeat each day. This also helps to prevent infection.
- It is common to feel many mixed emotions after the birth. Postnatal depression can be helped by the use of uplifting and comforting oils, such as lavender, bergamot, jasmine, rose and neroli. Geranium and clary sage can help to normalise hormonal imbalance and regulate mood swings. Use in the bath, for massage or in vaporisers.
- Engorged breasts can be soothed using a cold compress, or through gentle massage, using 2–3 drops each of juniper, lemon and fennel seed oil to 1 tablespoon (15 ml) of base oil or cream.

- For sore nipples, blend 1 drop each of rose or geranium, sandalwood and lavender in 1 teaspoon (5 ml) of non-oily cream or gel between feeds. Wipe off using a bland cream before each feed or use squeezed lemon peel for wiping nipples.

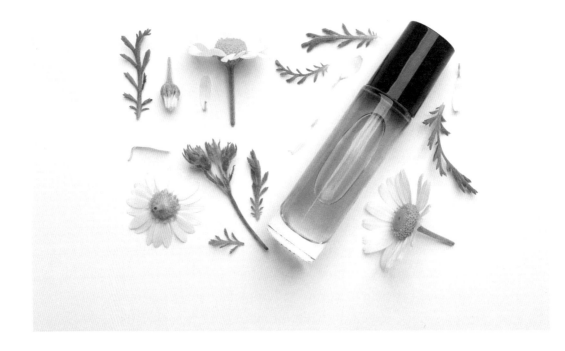

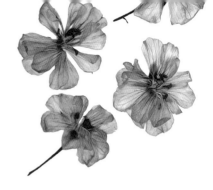

CHILDREN

BABIES AND YOUNG CHILDREN

Babies and young children respond especially well to natural healing methods, but their extra sensitivity must be taken into account. Do not attempt to substitute a home remedy for professional treatment if it is needed.

0–12 months: Use 1 drop only of either lavender, rose, Roman chamomile or geranium essential oil, diluted in 1 teaspoon carrier oil for massage or bathing.

1–5 years: Use only 2–3 drops of the 'safe' essential oils as above, diluted in 1 teaspoon carrier oil for massage or bathing; avoid all those oils that are potentially toxic or may cause skin irritation. (See Safety guidelines, page 185, for which oils to avoid.)

OLDER CHILDREN

Older children enjoy the stimulation of different scents. By the age of six they can recognise a wide range of smells, and enjoy being introduced to new experiences. It is fun to choose an oil to put in the bath or use as a scent. Geranium and lavender are popular with children because they are familiar and sweet. Add about 5 drops to the bath at bedtime.

6–12 years: Use as for adults but in half the stated concentration.

13 plus: Use as directed for adults.

COMMON CHILDHOOD COMPLAINTS

Many common childhood complaints can be treated with essential oils. Always check the dilution with the guidelines above.

- Nappy rash in babies and infants can be prevented by regular bathing using 1 drop of either lavender or Roman chamomile diluted in 1 teaspoon (5 ml) of carrier oil. If nappy rash does occur, add 1 drop each of lavender or Roman/German chamomile to 1 teaspoon (5 ml) of a non/greasy baby cream and apply gently at each nappy change: Nappy rash is often caused by thrush.

- Restlessness and insomnia in babies, infants and older children can be helped by the use of lavender, rose, Roman chamomile or ylang ylang in the bath or for massage. Alternatively, use a vaporiser in the bedroom (ensure it is out of children's reach), or put 1 or 2 drops of oil on the pillow or pajamas.

- Tummy ache and colic in babies, infants and older children can be eased by 2 drops each of lavender, marjoram, fennel seed and Roman chamomile in 1 teaspoon (5 ml) of carrier oil gently massaged to the lower back or stomach in a clockwise direction.

- Teething pain in babies and infants can be relieved by mixing 1 drop each of Roman chamomile and lavender in 1 teaspoon (5 ml) of carrier oil and massaging into the cheek.

- For cuts, spots, insect bites and other skin blemishes for children over 12 months old, apply 1 drop of neat lavender.

INFECTIOUS ILLNESSES

The most useful oils for stimulating the immune system and fighting viruses of all kinds in children, including flu, chickenpox and measles, are frankincense, geranium, lavender and tea-tree. A few drops of these oils should be used in a vaporiser or put on the pillow or on a tissue for use throughout the day and night.

- For fever and whooping cough, add a few drops of holy basil and bergamot to a vaporiser or a dish of steaming water in the sickroom. Steam vaporisation is especially useful during whooping cough to help relieve coughing.

- Colds and coughs in babies and older children respond well to the use of essential oils. Put 1 or 2 drops each of holy basil, marjoram, eucalyptus and tea-tree on the pillow or pajamas. You can also mix 3 drops of this combination to 1 teaspoon (5 ml) of olive oil. Alternatively, use a few drops of any of the above oils in a vaporiser in the bedroom (ensure it is well out of reach).

- For babies and children, add 2–4 drops of lavender and holy basil to the bath at the first signs of a cold developing.

- To help reduce itching and prevent scarring from chickenpox, make a lotion using 50 ml of witch-hazel and 50 ml of rosewater, with 2 drops each of German/Roman chamomile, tea-tree and lavender and dab onto the blisters. If the child is under five, add up to 3 drops of lavender or Roman chamomile to a warm bath and soak for 10 minutes at least twice a day.

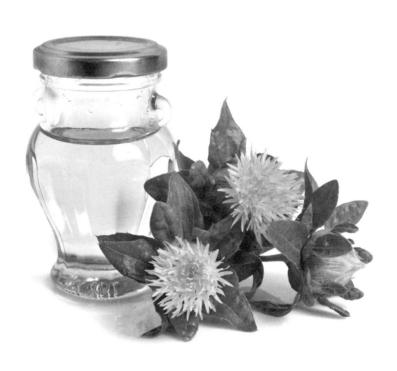

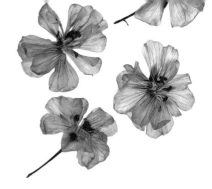

SKIN CONDITIONS

ABSCESSES AND BOILS

These often occur when the body is exhausted or rundown, at times of hormonal upheaval, and especially if the person is on a poor diet. Always keep the area clean and treat a boil or abscess before it bursts to avoid the spread of infection.

- Make up a hot compress using clean lint with 2 drops each of tea-tree and lavender, apply to the affected area; then treat it with a combination of 1 drop each of neat lavender and tea-tree at least 3 times daily, if possible. Cover with a plaster only if necessary.
- A green clay dressing with 1 drop of tea-tree may also be used to help draw out the pus.
- 5–10 drops of an antiseptic essential oil can be added to the bath, such as German chamomile, geranium, juniper, lavender and tea-tree.

ACNE

See page **229**.

ATHLETE'S FOOT AND RINGWORM

These are both contagious fungal infections characterised by red, flaky skin and itching. Athlete's foot occurs between the toes, sometimes affecting the toe nails. Ringworm shows on the skin as distinct red rings. It generally affects the scalp, knees, elbows or between the fingers. Let the skin breathe by avoiding tight clothes and nylon socks.

- Make a blend using 1 teaspoon (5 ml) of almond oil and 1 drop each of lavender, oregano and tea-tree, and apply at least 3 times a day. Tea-tree may also be applied neat (or diluted in a gel) – check sensitisation first by patch test.
- A few drops of the above oils may also be added to the bath, or to a footbath in the case of athlete's foot.

BEAUTY, SKIN AND HAIR CARE

For a detailed guide to caring for all parts of your body, including (ageing) skin, the face, breasts, eyes, hair, nail care and more, see Part III.

CHILBLAINS

Frostbite and chilblains are well-known injuries from cold. While frostbite causes acute tissue necrosis of the fingers, toes, nose and ears (rarely elsewhere), chilblains mostly affect the elderly with sedentary lifestyles. Women are more likely to develop chilblains than men. They occur at the extremities of the body – fingers and toes mainly – due to cold and lack of circulation. Exercise and warm clothing are important preventative factors. For chilblains:

- Apply ginger and tea-tree essential oils neat (or diluted in a gel) to the affected area.
- Local blood circulation can be improved by massaging the feet or hands with 2 drops of marjoram, 1 drop of ginger and 1 drop of black pepper in 1 teaspoon (5 ml) of carrier oil.

COLD SORES AND HERPES

Cold sores, also called fever blisters, can show up anywhere on your body. They're most likely to appear on the outside of your mouth and lips, but you can also find them on your nose and cheeks. **Cold sores** are caused by the **herpes** simplex virus. There are two types of the **herpes** simplex virus: type 1 (HSV-1) causes cold sores, and type 2 (HSV-2) causes genital herpes. Sometimes people confuse cold sores with genital herpes. Cold sores are also contagious, since they are viral infections, however they do resolve by themselves in 2–4 weeks.

Mix 3 drops each of tea-tree, frankincense, eucalyptus and lemon oil with 2 tablespoons (30 ml) of gel or jojoba oil and apply several times daily as soon as the first signs occur.

ECZEMA (ATOPIC DERMATITIS) AND PSORIASIS

This type of skin condition is characterised by flaky skin, itchy rashes, inflammation and sometimes weeping blisters or scabs. It is frequently associated with hereditary allergic tendencies, but often flares up during times of emotional difficulties or stress. It is important to try to locate the cause of the problem and deal with it directly. This means identifying the type of allergens that aggravate the condition and avoiding them (these may be particular household chemicals, dust, or certain foods); it may also mean looking at the emotional environment and making changes if necessary.

- In general, the most useful oils for **eczema** are German chamomile, juniper and tea-tree, and the best medium is usually a non-allergenic, light, aqueous (water-based) cream or gel. You can also add about 6 drops of tea-tree and German chamomile to 1 tablespoon (15 ml) of cream or gel to make a very dilute ointment, and apply at least 3 times daily.
- If the condition is weepy or inflamed, 2 drops of myrrh or patchouli should be included in the above cream or gel.

- If the condition is very itchy, add a few drops of German chamomile, tea-tree and juniper to a cold compress and apply to the skin. Using a few drops of chamomile or lavender in the bath can also help to alleviate itching. (A handful of powdered or colloidal oatmeal, available from some chemists, is also very soothing when added to the bathwater.)

- Since eczema takes many forms and is often stress-related, it is helpful to try to ease emotional tension by using relaxing and uplifting oils such as lavender, geranium, bergamot, neroli or rose for general use in the bath or as room fragrances.

- Some of my naturopath colleagues recommend application (twice daily) of your own urine on the affected area for at least 15 minutes before washing it off. According to them, it is quite effective for treating chronic skin conditions like eczema and psoriasis. I have seen dramatic improvement in condition with some of my clients also. Follow with an application of essential oils.

- Sometimes confused with eczema, **psoriasis** is a common, genetically determined inflammatory skin disorder of unknown cause. Dry, thick and raised patches on the **skin** are the most common sign of **psoriasis**. These patches are often covered with a silvery-white coating called scale, and they tend to itch. Psoriasis is not an infection of the skin and therefore not contagious, so touching the affected skin and then touching someone else will not transmit the condition. **Psoriasis** typically affects the outside of the elbows, knees or scalp, though it can appear on any location, I have seen it on almost all the parts of the body. Useful oils are cade, juniper, benzoin, frankincense, tea-tree and patchouli. Add 10 drops of any three of these oils in 1 teaspoon (5 ml) of jojoba oil for skin application.

- Both eczema and psoriasis can be helped greatly with evening primrose oil taken orally. (See Appendix 1, page **323**.)

VARICOSE VEINS AND PILES (HAEMORRHOIDS)

These conditions are both caused by dilated veins brought on by poor circulation and are especially common during pregnancy. Varicose veins occur mainly in the legs; piles (haemorrhoids) around the anal area. They both require similar treatments, although sufferers from varicose veins need more patience to see any improvement. The following treatments should be carried out in addition to gentle exercise (inverted yoga postures are especially helpful), keeping weight off the feet as much as possible, improving your diet and losing weight.

- The most useful oils are cypress, juniper and geranium: use 5–10 drops of the combination in a sitz bath. Other oils of benefit to use in the bath include lavender, juniper and rosemary.
- To make an oil that will both prevent and alleviate varicose veins, mix 4 drops of geranium and 4 drops of cypress with 1 tablespoon (15 ml) of carrier oil (or add to a non-greasy cream). Then use the oil blend to stroke the legs very gently, working upwards from the ankle to thigh (do not massage directly on the veins themselves).
- To treat piles, make an ointment by adding 2 drops of myrtle or cypress to 1 teaspoon (5 ml) of gel or jojoba oil, and rub around the anal area as required.

VERRUCA, WARTS AND CORNS

For these conditions, put a single drop of neat tea-tree on the centre of the verruca, wart or corn every morning and cover with a plaster. It may take several weeks to see any result, but it is effective in the long run. You can also use a combination of 15 drops each of tea-tree with oregano in 1 teaspoon (5 ml) of calendula oil. Apply 3 times daily to the affected area.

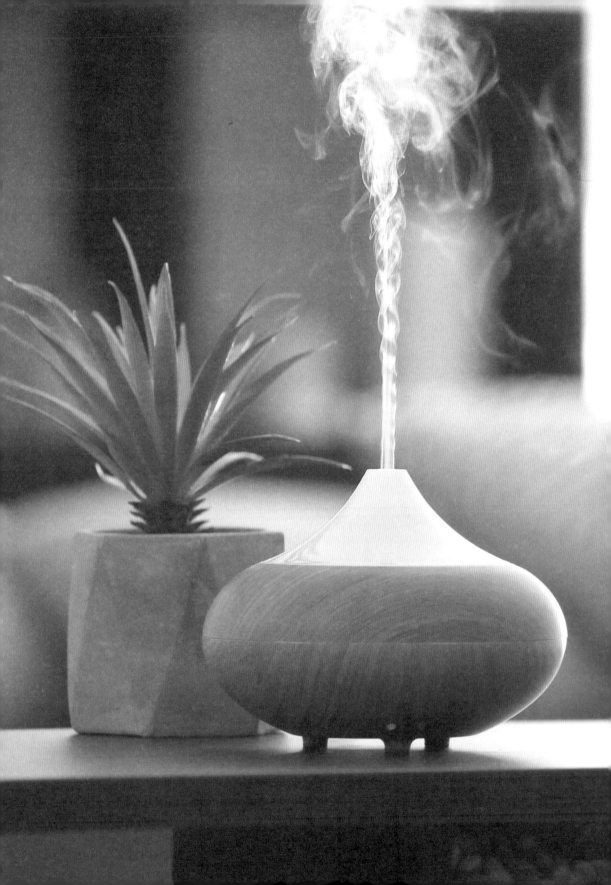

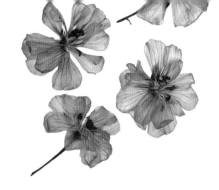

APPENDIXES

APPENDIX 1

NATURE'S GIFT: EVENING PRIMROSE OIL

A panacea for modern ailments

Ever since I came to know of evening primrose oil and its multiple benefits, I have wondered how a single plant oil can be so versatile in its effects. Once I understood the way it works on the body, my doubts were cleared to quite an extent and I was willing to try the product. I was amazed at the results reported to me by clients. Out of my experience, I now can safely recommend intake of this oil (1 teaspoon/5 ml daily) to everybody, especially women 30-plus. It is best to ingest this oil daily for a period of three months, stop for six months then resume for three months, and repeat to experience the difference in your health and body energy level.

Evening primrose is not a primrose at all. Rather, it is a member of the rosebay willowherb (Onagraceae) family. It acquired its common name because of its bright yellow primrose-like flowers and because its flowers open between 6pm and 7pm, when eight to ten of the large, fragrant flowers burst open every minute. The flowers usually last for the whole of the next day in dull weather but will fade quickly in bright sunlight.

Unlike many other natural products, which are usually known for a therapeutic effect on a single condition, evening primrose oil has properties which make it useful for a very wide range of conditions, including blood pressure, gout, hiccups, breast problems, PMS, faulty blood vessels, brittle nails and a score of other ailments.

All these problems seem very different, but evening primrose contains an element needed in each one. Evening primrose oil is a rich source of essential fatty acids (EFA), also called vitamin F, which are required by the body but can't make them. They are an essential part of nutrition. It also contains a rare substance, gamma linolenic acid (GLA), which sets it apart from most other vegetable oils. Roughly 60 per cent of the brain is made up of lipids, of which an important part are EFA. They are vital for the proper growth and development of the brain and the central nervous system. Essential fatty acids have two major roles. First they are constituents of all cell membranes and all the tissues in the body; secondly they give rise to highly reactive molecules, the prostaglandins and leukotrienes.

GLA is very special in its function. Firstly it helps build healthy cell membranes in every single cell of the body and secondly, GLA converts, inside the body, to a physiologically active substance called prostaglandin E1 (PGE1). GLA and PGE1 together provided by evening primrose oil are what make this oil so useful for restoring the balance of the body system and treating a wide range of disorders.

The fatty acids are an essential part of nutrition and perform all kinds of vital functions within the body:

- they give energy
- they help maintain body temperature
- they insulate the nerves
- They cushion and protect tissues

- They are part of the structure of every cell in our body and are vital for metabolism
- They are precursors of the all-important short lived regulating molecules, the **prostaglandins**.

Prostaglandins were discovered by Swedish scientist Ulf von Euler in the 1930s. He first found these molecules in seminal fluid and thought they came from the prostate gland, however, later scientists discovered that they can be found throughout the body. Prostaglandins have been found particularly in blood vessel walls, macrophages, platelets, duodenal secretions, nerves and every organ. They have an extremely short lifespan and most are removed from the blood during single passage through the lungs. They are naturally unstable because they have highly efficient mechanisms that break them down. The very short lifespan of prostaglandins makes them difficult to administer as drugs, since they have to be given intravenously.

Prostaglandins act as vital cell regulators. They control every cell and every organ in your body on a second-by-second basis. The nearest thing to them is hormones, which also have an important messenger role.

There are three series of prostaglandins, PG1, PG2, and PG3. Each of these has a different chemical structure and within each series there are different types classified by the letters A, B, D, E, F, etc. In all, there are at least 50 different prostaglandins and still new ones being discovered.

The three series of prostaglandins are each derived from a different fatty acid. Series 1 and 2 both come from the linoleic acid family. Series 3 is derived from eicosapentaenoic acid (EPA), a member of the alpha-linolenic acid family and most commonly found in oily seafoods.

Each prostaglandin has a different role to play, and health problems can arise when the different series of prostaglandins are out of balance with each other. The balance between the 1 and 2 series PGs can be influenced by diet. In inflammatory conditions, the end products of arachidonic acid metabolism – prostaglandins series 2, cyclo-oxygenase and thromboxane

A2 – are being produced in too great a quantity, whereas not enough PGE 1 is being produced.

Two of the most widely used drugs, steroids and non-steroidal anti-inflammatory drugs (NSAIDs) work by inhibiting the biosynthesis of prostaglandins. By suppressing the production of prostaglandins, the drugs dampen down inflammation. However, the trouble with this drug approach is that all the prostaglandins are knocked out, including the good ones. Evening primrose oil works in a completely different way from these powerful drugs. Instead of stopping the manufacture of prostaglandins, evening primrose goes on to make the anti-inflammatory prostaglandin E1, so manipulates the prostaglandins in a natural way.

PROSTAGLANDIN E1 (PGE1) seems to have the most desirable qualities among all the prostaglandins and evening primrose oil is easily converted to prostaglandin E1. The benefits of PGE1 include:

- It promotes dilation of blood vessels
- It lowers arterial pressure
- It inhibits thrombosis
- It inhibits cholesterol synthesis
- It inhibits inflammation and controls arthritis
- It inhibits abnormal cell proliferation
- It inhibits platelet aggregation
- It regulates production of saliva and tears
- It elevates cyclic AMP (adenosine monophosphate).

Given these benefits, evening primrose oil is useful for a wide range of symptoms.

PMS (PREMENSTRUAL SYNDROME)

PMS is a condition which affects the whole system. It can cause havoc in women's lives, at worst wrecking relationships, marriages and careers. Six of the most common symptoms experienced by women with PMS are irritability, depression, breast pain, bloating, headaches and clumsiness. However, the cluster of symptoms include on the physical side: swollen ankles, legs, reduced libido, constipation, hot flushes, backache, nausea, acne, cramps, food cravings, lethargy and fatigue; and on the psychological/emotional side: anxiety, mood swings, suicidal impulses, low self-esteem, weeping for no obvious reason, sudden tantrums, lack of concentration and lapses of memory.

Evening primrose oil has been used successfully as part of a treatment program for PMS since the beginning of 1980s. Trials have consistently proved that more than 80 per cent of women who suffer from PMS improve on evening primrose oil.

Women suffering from PMS are thought to be low on essential fatty acids and also considered to be low in the important prostaglandin E1 made from EFAs. They also have an imbalance of the various prostaglandins. A shortage of EFAs can lead to an apparent excess of the female hormone prolactin. Prolactin produces changes in mood and fluid metabolism, similar to those found in PMS. It is thought that GLA and PGE1, derived from evening primrose oil, can damp down these effects of prolactin and other hormones.

Though evening primrose oil has an important role to play as nutritional therapy for PMS, other important considerations are diet, specific minerals and vitamin supplements, exercise, and lifestyle changes to reduce stress. The various vitamins and minerals found useful in controlling PMS are vitamin C (between 500 mg to 3 g per day), B complex tablets (appropriate ratio), vitamin B6 (50 mg per day) and zinc (10 mg a day).

The most suitable dose of evening primrose oil is 1 teaspoon (5 ml) per day or a minimum of two capsules three times a day after meals. Though ingestion of the liquid may not be palatable to some it may be a preferable option to avoid the extra gelatin.

FIBROCYSTIC BREAST CONDITION AND BREAST PAIN (MASTALGIA)

Breast pain is common in women and can be associated with the menstrual cycle. It can occur as part of PMS, in some cases lasting as long as 2 weeks in every 4. Or it may have nothing to do with a woman's menstrual cycle. In such cases the pain may be continuous, resulting in the sufferer feeling irritable and depressed. Typically, the breasts feel heavy and tender, with a lumpy granular texture. Many women with these symptoms may visit their doctor fearing breast cancer.

It is believed that the breast pain is caused by abnormal sensitivity of breast tissue to normal levels of the hormones prolactin and oestrogen and congestion of axillary lymph nodes. Until recently breast pain has been treated with hormone-related drugs which have their own side effects; **however, evening primrose oil is an effective alternative with none of the side effects.**

There is an interesting relationship between heart disease in men and mastalgia and PMS in women. In both the cases, it is the congestion of axillary lymph nodes that is the cause. In women, congestion of axillary lymph nodes leads to congestion of lymph in and around the breast area, causing mastalgia. In men, the congestion of axillary lymph nodes over a period of time leads to arterial blockages, ultimately resulting in coronory heart disease. In societies where there is a high rate of death from heart disease among young and middle-aged men, there is a correspondingly high rate of breast disease and PMS in young and middle-aged women.

If a high intake of saturated fat is associated with benign breast disease and other diseases, then increasing the intake of polyunsaturated fatty acids (PUFAs) may reverse or prevent the development of mastalgia and PMS. Women with breast disease tend to have high rates of sebum production, which is a marker of EFA deficiency.

Evening primrose oil is useful as a treatment for breast pain because PGE1 can dampen down the effects of prolactin, may prevent the development of cysts and can help remove lumpiness in the breasts.

Women with breast pain have been found to have normal or near normal levels of linoleic acid. However, they have abnormally low levels of metabolites of linoleic acid, indicating they cannot metabolise it efficiently. Evening primrose oil works because its active ingredient is GLA, which bypasses the metabolic block. So the level of essential fatty acids is brought up to normal.

DIABETES

Even when diabetes is well controlled by insulin and diet, there can still be complications. Diabetes can lead to severe damage to the heart and circulation, to the eyes, to the kidneys and to nerves. The damage to the nerves – known medically as diabetic neuropathy – can lead to lots of skin problems, muscle weakness, bladder and intestinal problems, and impotence in men. Diabetic neuropathy affects about half of all diabetics and there has been no effective treatment for it.

Another common complication for diabetics is degeneration of the retina of the eye – diabetic retinopathy. This is a common cause of blindness in middle-aged people. This happens because diabetes causes swellings in the walls of the arteries feeding the retina and twists in the retinal veins. As a result, there are tiny hemorrhages and the retinal tissue degenerates and dies.

Evening primrose oil is a major breakthrough in the treatment of diabetic neuropathy. It has been found that evening primrose can actually reverse the nerve damage in diabetics. Recent research from scientists from France and Australia has provided evidence that diabetics cannot make GLA normally from linoleic acid in their diet and this inability to make GLA may be a cause of some of the long-term complications of diabetes. But GLA given to diabetics with nerve damage can both prevent and reverse diabetic nerve damage.

It has also been found useful to take evening primrose oil to prevent damage to the retina. There have been successful trials in Holland where linoleic acid was used, and it was found that the patients with diabetes who took large amounts of linoleic acid prevented the retinas from degenerating. Evening primrose oil works in the same way as linoleic acid, but because it is more powerful, you would not need to take as much. Dutch researchers have found that diabetic patients who are on a diet high in linoleic acid needed less insulin.

HEART DISEASE, VASCULAR DISORDERS AND HIGH BLOOD PRESSURE

Heart disease and diseases of the blood vessels are among the biggest killers. Despite a certain amount of controversy over the underlying risk factors that contribute to coronary deaths, a number are broadly accepted:

- High cholesterol level in blood
- Platelets that stick together unduly (platelet aggregation)
- High blood pressure
- Atheroma clogging up blood vessels
- Vascular spasm.

Ever since the 1950s, it has been known that linoleic acid is able to reduce cholesterol levels, but it means taking large quantities of linolenic acid, which would be very high in calories as well as relatively unpalatable. However it has since been realised that the power to reduce cholesterol levels is not so much vested in the linoleic acid itself, but in its metabolites dihomo-gammalinolenic acid (DGLA) and also arachidonic acid.

There is a strong association between the incidence of cardiovascular disease and reduced levels of DGLA. In the metabolic pathway of linoleic acid, DGLA is formed from gamma linolenic acid (GLA), the active ingredient of evening primrose oil. So you need to take only a small dose of evening primrose oil and it will be more potent than linoleic acid in reducing cholesterol. The recommended dose is approximately 5 mg per day.

Evening primrose oil has an interesting effect on cholesterol levels. It will only bring down cholesterol levels if they are high, but it will have no effect on cholesterol levels if they are normal or low. This is because evening primrose oil works physiologically to regulate cholesterol metabolism instead of working pharmacologically as a drug.

Like other polyunsaturated fatty acids (PUFAs), evening primrose oil either has no effect on HDL (high density lipoprotein) cholesterol or actually increases it. The cholesterol-lowering action of evening primrose oil is entirely because it is able to lower the harmful LDL (low density lipoprotein) cholesterol. Lowering LDL cholesterol reduces the risk of heart attack. HDL cholesterol is desirable because it actually helps to transport cholesterol away from places where it may be harmful. **Evening primrose oil has the very beneficial effect of raising the HDL/LDL ratio.**

The clotting agents in blood are called platelets. A risk factor for cardiovascular disorders occurs when the platelets in blood aggregate abnormally (they bunch up and stick together). Evening primrose oil is very effective in stopping this process.

When platelets stick to cholesterol deposits this quickly leads to a clot, which can block the flow of blood. When a blood clot forms in an artery or a vein it is called a thrombosis. This blocks the circulation in the area. A clot in a coronary artery is a coronary thrombosis. In the brain it's a stroke. **Evening primrose oil helps because the GLA in evening primrose oil easily converts to DGLA, which is known to be able to reduce platelet aggregation. As well, evening primrose oil converts to prostaglandin E1 and PGE 1 is one of the most potent known inhibitors of platelet aggregation.**

People with high blood pressure run a greater risk of experiencing arteriosclerosis, heart failure, stroke and kidney disease. Evening primrose oil has been considered more effective in lowering blood pressure than much higher doses of other polyunsaturated fatty acids. Diets rich in PUFAs may not only arrest the progression of atheroma, but may actually reverse it, allowing the obstruction to be cleared. **Taking evening primrose oil as supplement would be worthwhile even for those people whose cardiovascular system is already damaged.**

CANCER

Research in South Africa (published in the *South African Medical Journal*) showed that **gamma linolenic acid, taken from evening primrose oil, reduced cancer cell growth up to 70 per cent.** Six different laboratories in 4 different countries have since obtained similar results, finding that PUFAs normalise human cancer cells. The tests were conducted on at least nine different human malignant cell lines, including cancers of the liver, bone, oesophagus, breast, prostate and skin. In all these tests, the normal cells remain unaffected.

What researchers observed is that the GLA in evening primrose oil may be working in three different way:.

1. Lipid peroxides: When human cancer cells are exposed to polyunsaturated fatty acids in the laboratory, the cells generate large amounts of substances called lipid peroxides and die. Several PUFAs have been tried and GLA seems to be the best – it is highly toxic to malignant cells, but has no toxic effects whatsoever on the normal cells.

2. It bypasses the delta-6-desaturase enzyme block. Cancer is a known blocking agent of the metabolic pathway of linoleic acid. This block occurs at the first step, between linoleic acid and gamma linolenic acid, by inhibiting the delta-6-desaturase enzyme. GLA in evening primrose oil by-passes this block by starting at the second stage in the metabolic pathway. This means that GLAQ can convert to DGLA and then to prostaglandin E1 without hindrance.

3. Prostaglandins: another way in which polyunsaturated fatty acids might be controlling cancer cells is by being converted into prostaglandins. Prostaglandins derived from PUFAs may inhibit the proliferation of human and animal tumour cells, and reverse transformed cells.

The use of evening primrose oil in the treatment of cancer aims to prevent cancerous cells from proliferating without affecting healthy cells. Orthodox treatment uses chemotherapy or radiation, which are toxic to cancerous as well as healthy cells, with unpleasant side effects. Since the findings of evening primrose oil are mostly subjective and not conclusive, some therapists may have their doubts. However, evening primrose oil works more at a physiological level as a nutritional supplement without any side effects, which should be good reason to use it, as it will also help controlling the side effects of orthodox treatments like chemotherapy and radiation.

AIDS, VIRAL INFECTIONS AND POST-VIRAL FATIGUE

The most exciting development with evening primrose oil in recent years is its effect on viral infections. This could herald a radically new low-risk approach to treating viral infections including AIDS. Essential fatty acids are particularly important because they have direct virus-killing effects and are lethal to many viruses at surprisingly low concentrations. They are also required for the antiviral actions of the body's own natural virus fighter, interferon.

But in order to be effective as an antiviral agent, interferon needs prostaglandins, which are converted from essential fatty acids. Without prostaglandins, the antiviral actions of interferon are lost or certainly much diminished.

It is now known that essential fatty acids are severely depleted with AIDS and reduced in patients with glandular fever and other viral infections. This may be caused by the effects of the virus itself rather than any lack of essential fatty acids in the diet. The rationale for giving evening primrose oil is to increase the supply of the metabolites of the parent EFAs so that the EFAs can do their virus-killing work and also help interferon do its virus-fighting job.

ECZEMA (ATOPIC DERMATITIS)

As long ago as the 1930s it was known that essential fatty acids are vital for healthy skin and hair. But it was only in the 1990s that people realised the efficacy of evening primrose oil on skin disorders, especially eczema. Studies have found that whenever there are low levels of essential fatty acids:

- The skin becomes scaly, rough and sheds dandruff-like scales. In severe deficiency, an eczema-like dermatitis may develop and the skin may break down
- Wounds take longer to heal
- There is greater water loss from the skin, making it drier and age more quickly.

Eczema is chronic, patchy, mild inflammation of the surface of the skin, which almost always begins in infancy or early childhood. It can be made worse by irritants, but often occurs without any apparent cause. In recent years, evening primrose oil has had excellent results in the treatment of eczema, in both adults and children.

All studies done so far agree that people with eczema have below-normal levels of GLA, DGLA, AA, PGE1 and metabolites of alpha linolenic acid. The enzyme delta-6-desaturase is needed to get from linoleic acid to the next step and from alpha linolenic acid to the next step.

Evening primrose oil completely bypasses this enzyme block by starting at the next stage in the metabolic pathway of the linoleic acid family. Please note that the improvement does not happen overnight: it takes 4 to 12 weeks after starting ingestion of evening primrose oil.

ASTHMA, HAYFEVER, ALLERGIES AND OTHER ATOPIC CONDITIONS

On the face of it, eczema, asthma, hayfever and allergies all sound like very different conditions but in fact they have a lot in common: they are all to do with a weak immune system and an abnormal body defence mechanism called atopy. Atopy, or a generalised allergic response, can show itself as any or all of a variety of conditions.

Eczema is closely linked with other atopic conditions like asthma and hayfever, and it is also common to find other members of the family suffering from these conditions. It has long been known that people with eczema, asthma and allergies have something wrong with their immune systems, mainly due to a fatty acids abnormality that affects various other parts regulating the immune system, particularly PGE1 and T lymphocytes.

Evening primrose oil helps to correct the faulty immune system in people with atopic conditions, as it converts to PGE1, which stimulates the T- lymphocytes playing an all important role in the immune system.

HYPERACTIVE CHILDREN

It seems evening primrose oil works especially well on atopic children with a family history of such ailments as eczema, asthma, allergies, hayfever or migraine. The mothers of hyperactive children are often found to suffer from migraine, premenstrual tension or postnatal depression. **Evening primrose oil has helped to improve dramatically the lives of countless children and their families.** When combined with a nutritional and dietary approach, evening primrose oil work wonders on hyperactive children. The key things to take out of the child's diet are artificial colouring, flavouring and preservatives.

Hyperactive children might be deficient in PGE1, which helps control the immune system and has an influence on such things like asthma, behaviour and thirst (via the kidneys). Salicylates, in aspirin and even in seemingly innocent foods as apples, oranges, peaches, strawberries, grapes, cherries, almonds and cucumbers are also known to block the formation of prostaglandins, therefore should be excluded from the diet. Parents are advised to give children only fresh foods and avoid anything with added vitamin E, however other vitamins and mineral supplements are very helpful since hyperactive children are found to be very low in zinc and magnesium. So evening primrose oil should be taken with its cofactors, which are zinc, vitamin B6, nicotinamide (vitamin B3) and vitamin C.

RHEUMATOID ARTHRITIS

Rheumatoid arthritis is the inflammatory form of arthritis, a chronic condition affecting connective tissues, mainly of joints, and can be very painful. Studies show using evening primrose oil by itself or using it along with fish oil have provided substantial improvement in their conditions and helped them reduce or give up treatment with conventional anti-inflammatory drugs. However, as yet there is no evidence that they act as agents which actually modify the disease.

SKIN, HAIR, EYES, NAILS AND BUST

The two major essential fatty acids, linoleic acid and gamma linolenic acid (GLA), in which evening primrose oil is rich, are natural skin nutrients. Linoleic acid and GLA are vital components of the structure of all cell membranes and are normally converted by the body into prostaglandins. Prostaglandins play an important role in maintaining skin health.

When evening primrose oil is applied directly to the skin, linoleic acid and GLA have a profound effect on reducing trans-epidermal water loss, therefore acting as a natural moisturiser and helping to slow down the ageing process.

The discovery that evening primrose oil can cure brittle nails was by chance. A medical trial was being conducted in Scotland using evening primrose oil for two conditions which make the eyes and mouth dry and painful (Sjogren syndrome and sicca syndrome). It was found that not only did the participants' dry eyes and mouths get better, but their brittle nails dramatically improved at the same time.

An unforeseen side effect of evening primrose oil in some women who have consumed evening primrose oil over a long period is increased bust size; however they noticed that they had not put on weight anywhere else in the body.

It has been observed that animals deprived of essential fatty acids suffered loss of their fur as well as dandruff-like conditions. Use of evening primrose oil has improved chronic dandruff and controlled hair loss.

SIDE EFFECTS

Though there are no noticeable side effects of evening primrose oil being used in capsule form or ingested directly as liquid, there are reports of seizures with the use of evening primrose oil. People at risk of seizures should avoid using it. Evening primrose oil lowers blood pressure in animals, but effects in humans are not clear. Headache, stomach pain, nausea and loose stools may occur.

RECOMMENDATION

It is recommended to consume cold-pressed evening primrose oil from a trusted source (manufacturer or repacker) and under the guidance of a therapist or practitioner. At Aromatantra, we repack our evening primrose after ensuring the quality and percentage of GLA available in the oil, and no synthetic preservatives or flavouring agents are added. The oil is available through mail order. Visit www.aromatantra.com

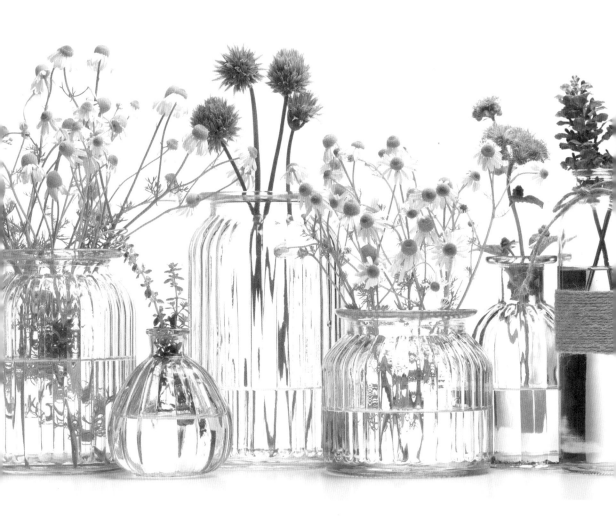

APPENDIX 2

READY REFERENCE:
THE THERAPEUTIC USES
OF ESSENTIAL OILS

This list has been compiled from the most reliable references available, as well as the author's own experience. **Bold** type indicates the oils commonly used in connection with the particular ailment.

ABDOMINAL CRAMP: Aniseed; **basil**; bergamot; caraway; chamomile, Roman; clove bud; fennel; lavender; **marjoram**, sweet; **melissa**, **true**; nutmeg; orange, bitter

ABSCESSES, BOILS: Cajuput; **chamomile, German**; clove bud; geranium; juniper berry; helichrysm; lavender; **lemon**; **niaouli**; palmarosa; **tea-tree** (infection); **thyme, red** (infection); **thyme, sweet**

ACNE: Bergamot; cajuput; **cedarwood**; **chamomile, German**; eucalyptus; **geranium**; helichrysm; **juniper berry**; **lavender**; lemon; neroli; palmarosa; patchouli; petitgrain; rosemary; sandalwood; **tea-tree**

AIR DISINFECTANT: **Basil**; **citronella**; **eucalyptus**; grapefruit; lemon; **lemongrass**; melissa; pine; rosemary; sage; thyme

ALLERGIES/SENSITIVE SKIN: Basil, holy; **chamomile, German**; clary sage; neroli; eucalyptus; grapefruit; hyssop; **lavender**; patchouli; sandalwood

ANTI-AGEING: Clary sage; **frankincense**; **geranium**; lavender; marjoram, sweet; **neroli**; orange, bitter; palmarosa; patchouli; rose otto; **sandalwood**; vetiver; ylang ylang

ANXIETY: **Basil**; bergamot; cedarwood; chamomile, Roman; **clary sage**; **geranium**; **lavender**; **lemon**; mandarin; **marjoram, sweet**; melissa; neroli; orange, sweet; patchouli; petitgrain; rose otto; rosemary; rosewood;

sandalwood; thyme; vetiver; ylang ylang

APPETITE, LACK OF: Bergamot; dill seed; chamomile, Roman; **coriander**; fennel; mandarin; oregano

ARTHRITIS: **Basil**; **black pepper**; **cajuput**; **clove**; chamomile, German; coriander; cypress; eucalyptus; **juniper**; lavandin; **lavender**; marjoram, sweet; niaouli; rosemary; sage; savory; thyme, sweet; **wintergreen**

ASTHMA: **Aniseed**; basil; bergamot; **cajuput**; cedarwood; chamomile, Roman; **eucalyptus**; frankincense; **hyssop**; lavender; lemon; mandarin; marjoram; neroli; niaouli; **pine**; **peppermint**; rose otto; rosemary; sage; thyme, sweet

BAD BREATH: Basil; bergamot; caraway; fennel seed; grapefruit; lemon; myrrh; nutmeg; orange, bitter; peppermint; spearmint; thyme, sweet

BEDWETTING: Cypress; mandarin; orange; pine; rosemary

BRONCHITIS: **Aniseed**; basil, holy; bay; black pepper; cajuput; cedarwood; clove bud; **cypress**; **eucalyptus**; frankincense; ginger; hyssop; juniper; **lavender**; lemon; sweet marjoram; myrrh; **niaouli**; **pine**; rose otto; rosemary; sage; sandalwood; tea-tree; thyme, red; thyme, sweet

BRUISES: Camphor; **chamomile, German**; fennel; helichrysm; **lavender**; lemon; **marjoram, sweet**; myrrh; rosemary; sage; tea-tree

BURNS: Benzoin; chamomile, German; **geranium**; helichrysm; **lavender**; palmarosa; rosewood; sage; tea-tree

CANDIDA (THRUSH): Bergamot; cinnamon bark; eucalyptus; geranium; juniper berry; oregano; rose otto; rosemary; **sage**; **tea-tree**; **thyme, sweet**

CATARRH: Basil, holy; benzoin; black pepper; **cajuput**; cedarwood; eucalyptus; lavender; lemon; **marjoram**; myrrh; **niaouli**; peppermint; rosemary; sage; sandalwood; tagetes; tea-tree

CELLULITE: Black pepper; cedarwood; cinnamon; cypress; **fennel**; geranium; grapefruit; juniper berry; lavender; **lemongrass**; **melissa**; patchouli; rosemary; sage; sandalwood

CIRRHOSIS: Clary sage; fennel seed; helichrysm; juniper; lavender; rosemary

CONSTIPATION: Aniseed; basil, holy; black pepper; chamomile, Roman; coriander; dill; fennel; ginger; juniper; mandarin; orange, bitter; **rosemary**

COUGHS AND COLDS: **Basil**; bay; **black pepper**; cedarwood; clove; **eucalyptus**; frankincense; geranium; juniper; lavender; lemon; marjoram; peppermint; pine; tea-tree; thyme, sweet

CRAMP: **Basil**; cajuput; chamomile, Roman; cypress; eucalyptus; **lavender**; mandarin; **marjoram, sweet**; rosemary; valerian

CUTS/WOUNDS: Benzoin; bergamot; camphor; cedarwood; **chamomile, German;** clove bud; cypress; eucalyptus; frankincense; **geranium;** hyssop; **lavender;** lemon; myrrh; **niaouli;** orange bitter; palmarosa; rose otto; rosemary; sage; tea-tree

CYSTITIS: Basil, sweet; bergamot; **cajuput;** chamomile, German; clove bud; coriander; eucalyptus; geranium; hyssop; **juniper; lavender;** niaouli; peppermint; **sandalwood;** thyme, red; thyme, sweet

DEBILITY: **Basil;** camphor; cinnamon bark; clove bud; coriander; geranium; hyssop; **lavandin; marjoram, sweet;** peppermint; pine; rosewood; savory; tea-tree; thyme, red; thyme, sweet; valerian

DEPRESSION: **Basil;** bergamot; chamomile; cinnamon bark; cypress; geranium; grapefruit; **hyssop; juniper; jasmine;** lemongrass; **melissa; neroli;** niaouli; orange; **petitgrain;** pine; rosemary; rose otto; rosewood; **sandalwood; vetiver; ylang ylang**

DERMATITIS: Benzoin; cade; cajuput; **chamomile, German; chamomile, Moroccan;** eucalyptus; **geranium;** hyssop; **juniper;** lavender; **lemon;** palmarosa; **patchouli;** rose otto; sage; tea-tree; thyme, sweet

DIABETES: clary sage; **eucalyptus;** geranium; juniper; **lemon;** pine; rosemary; thyme, sweet; **vetiver**

DIARRHOEA: Basil; black pepper; chamomile; cinnamon bark; clove bud; geranium; **ginger;** juniper; lemon; marjoram, sweet; myrrh; niaouli; nutmeg; **peppermint;** tea-tree; sandalwood; savory

EARACHE: Basil; cajuput; chamomile, Roman; lavender; rosemary; tea-tree

ECZEMA: Basil; **benzoin;** cajuput; **chamomile, German;** chamomile, Moroccan; clove bud; eucalyptus; frankincense; **geranium;** hyssop; **juniper; lavender;** myrrh; niaouli; **patchouli;** rose otto; sandalwood; tea-tree; thyme, sweet

EPILEPSY: Basil; cajuput; clary sage; lavender; marjoram, sweet; parsley leaf; rosemary; thyme, sweet

FLATULENCE: **Angelica; aniseed; basil;** bergamot; black pepper; **caraway; coriander; fennel;** ginger; lavender; mandarin; marjoram, sweet; niaouli; orange, bitter; **peppermint;** thyme, sweet

FLU: **Basil; cajuput;** clove bud; coriander; **eucalyptus;** lavender; **lemon;** lemongrass; myrrh; **niaouli;** peppermint; pine; rosemary; sage; tea-tree; **thyme, sweet**

FLUID RETENTION: Cedarwood; cypress; fennel; geranium; grapefruit; juniper berry; lemon; orange; pine; rosemary

FRIGIDITY: Aniseed; black pepper; clove; clary sage; chamomile, Moroccan; frankincense; **ginger; neroli**; rose otto; sandalwood; ylang ylang

FUNGAL INFECTIONS (SKIN): Cypress; geranium; lavender; niaouli; oregano; patchouli; pine; rosemary; sage; sandalwood; savory; tagetes; **tea-tree**; thyme, sweet

GASTRIC ULCERS: Basil; **chamomile, German**; fennel; **geranium**; lemon; lavender; marjoram, sweet; niaouli; oregano; tea-tree

GASTROENTERITIS: **Basil**; bergamot; **cajuput**; caraway; **chamomile, German**; chamomile, Moroccan; clove bud; coriander; cypress; fennel; **juniper berry**; lavender; lemongrass; mandarin, sweet; **niaouli**; nutmeg; patchouli; **peppermint**; sage; tea-tree; thyme

GINGIVITIS: Clary sage; juniper; lemon; sage

GLANDULAR: Clary sage; **geranium**; pine; rosemary

GOUT: Basil; Roman chamomile; fennel; **juniper**; lemon; pine; rosemary

GUM INFECTIONS (PYORRHOEA): Cinnamon bark; clove bud; cypress; geranium; juniper; rosemary; tea-tree

HAEMORRHOIDS: Bergamot; cajuput; **clary sage; cypress**; frankincense; geranium; myrrh; **neroli; niaouli**; patchouli; sandalwood; tea-tree; valerian

HEADACHE: **Basil**; chamomile, Roman; eucalyptus; **lavender**; lemon; **marjoram, sweet**; melissa, true; peppermint; rosemary

HEARTBURN: Chamomile, Moroccan and Roman; peppermint; sandalwood

HEPATITIS: Basil; clove bud; eucalyptus; juniper; lemongrass; myrrh; niaouli; petitgrain; rosemary

HERPES: Bergamot; eucalyptus; geranium; lavender; lemon; niaouli (genital); sage

HICCUPS: Mandarin

HIGH BLOOD PRESSURE: Basil, sweet; **clary sage**; Juniper; **lavender; lemon**; marjoram, sweet; ylang ylang

HYSTERIA: Lemongrass; melissa, true

IMPOTENCE: Aniseed; black pepper; cinnamon bark; **ginger**; peppermint; pine; rose otto; savory; thyme, sweet; **ylang ylang**

INDIGESTION: **Aniseed**; basil; bergamot; black pepper; caraway; coriander; dill; **fennel; ginger; lemon**; lemongrass; mandarin; melissa, true; orange, bitter; orange, sweet; **peppermint**; rosemary

INFLAMMATION: **Chamomile, German**; clary sage; frankincense; geranium; **lavender**; myrrh; peppermint; petitgrain; rose otto; sandalwood

INSECT BITES: Basil; cajuput; **lavender**; melissa, true; niaouli; sage; tea-tree;

thyme, sweet

INSECT REPELLENT: Basil; cedarwood; **citronella**; clove bud; **eucalyptus**; geranium; lemon; lemongrass; peppermint; thyme

INSOMNIA: Bergamot; chamomile, Roman; clary sage; cypress; geranium; lavender; mandarin; marjoram, sweet; melissa, true; neroli; orange, bitter; orange, sweet; rose otto; **sandalwood**; valerian; ylang ylang

IRRITATION (SKIN): Chamomile, German; cedarwood; lavender; neroli; peppermint; sandalwood

KIDNEY, GENERAL: Cedarwood; **fennel**; geranium; **juniper**; **lavender**; **lemon**; niaouli; pine; **sage**; sandalwood; thyme, red; thyme, sweet

KIDNEY INFECTIONS: Clove bud; coriander; myrrh; **sandalwood**; sage; savory; **thyme**

KIDNEY STONES: Fennel; geranium; hyssop; **juniper**; lemon

LABOUR PAIN: Clary sage; **fennel**; nutmeg

LARYNGITIS: Black pepper; cajuput; cypress; eucalyptus; **lemon**; **myrrh**; niaouli; peppermint; sage; **sandalwood**

LIVER SLUGGISH: Basil; black pepper; cajuput; **chamomile, Moroccan**; juniper; **lemon**; lemongrass; melissa, true; peppermint; **rosemary**; **thyme, sweet**; vetiver

LOW BLOOD PRESSURE: **Cinnamon**; clove bud; hyssop; **lemon**; neroli; peppermint; **rosemary**; sage; savory; thyme, sweet

LUMBAGO: Aniseed; eucalyptus; fennel; geranium; sandalwood

MENOPAUSE: Aniseed; basil; bergamot; chamomile, Roman; **clary sage**; cypress; **fennel**; geranium; hyssop; jasmine; juniper; lavender; lemon; mandarin; melissa, true; **peppermint**; pine; **rose otto**; rosemary; sage; sandalwood

MENTAL FATIGUE: **Basil**; cajuput; **clove bud**; coriander; juniper berry; lavender; **neroli**; **peppermint**; **rosemary**; rosewood

MIGRAINE: Aniseed; **basil**; chamomile, German; **eucalyptus**; **lavender**; marjoram, sweet; melissa, true; neroli; peppermint; rosemary

LACK OF MILK (BREAST FEEDING): Aniseed; dill; fennel

MOUTH ULCERS: Basil; clove bud; geranium; **juniper**; lemon; myrrh; niaouli; rose otto; sage; sandalwood; tea-tree

MUSCULAR PAIN: Bergamot; **black pepper**; camphor; cajuput; **cinnamon**; chamomile, German; **chamomile, Moroccan**; chamomile, Roman; eucalyptus; frankincense; **juniper**; **nutmeg**; **rosemary**; **thyme, sweet**;

vetiver

NAUSEA: Black pepper; caraway; fennel; ginger; mandarin; melissa, true; peppermint; sandalwood

NERVOUS EXHAUSTION: **Basil; clary sage;** clove bud; coriander; geranium; **lavender; savory;** tea-tree; thyme, sweet

NEURALGIA: Camphor; **Roman chamomile; clove bud; eucalyptus;** ginger; **juniper;** lavender; marjoram, sweet; **peppermint;** pine; rosemary; sandalwood

NEURITIS: Chamomile, German; chamomile, Roman; clary sage; clove; cypress; juniper; niaouli; thyme, sweet

OEDEMA: Cedarwood; cypress; eucalyptus; geranium; **juniper;** orange; patchouli; rosemary; sage; sandalwood

OSTEOPOROSIS: Eucalyptus; lavender; lemon; lemongrass; **rosemary;** sage

OVARIES: Clary sage; cypress; rosemary; sage; ylang ylang

PALPITATIONS: **Aniseed;** fennel; lavender; mandarin; melissa, true; neroli; petitgrain; rosemary; valerian; ylang ylang

PERIODS, LACK OF: Aniseed; chamomile, German; cinnamon bark; clary sage; fennel; juniper berry; peppermint; rosemary; sage; tagetes; thyme, sweet; vetiver

PERIODS, PAINFUL: Aniseed; basil (congestion); chamomile, German (congestion); clary sage; cypress (congestion); fennel; geranium (congestion); juniper; lavender; **marjoram, sweet;** peppermint; pine; sage (congestion)

PERIODS, SCANTY: Basil; **chamomile, Roman;** clary sage (hormonal); fennel; juniper; lavender; **melissa, true (hormonal);** rosemary; **rose otto** (hormonal); thyme, sweet

PERSPIRATION: Basil; cypress; geranium; lavender; neroli; sage

PREMENSTRUAL SYNDROME (PMS): Bergamot; chamomile, Roman; **clary sage;** geranium; lavender; melissa, true; rose otto; **neroli;** sage (congestion); sandalwood

PROSTATE, ENLARGED: Basil; caraway; cypress

PSORIASIS: Benzoin; bergamot; cajuput; chamomile, German; lavender; lemon; niaouli; sandalwood

RESPIRATORY INFECTION: Frankincense; **lemon; niaouli; petitgrain; pine;** rosewood; tagetes; thyme, red

RHEUMATISM: Bay; **basil;** black pepper; **cajuput;** camphor; clove bud;

eucalyptus; frankincense; geranium (inflammation); **ginger** (warming); hyssop; **juniper**; lavandin; **lavender**; lemongrass; **marjoram, sweet**; myrrh; niaouli; **nutmeg** (analgesic); petitgrain (nervous); pine; **rosemary** (stiffness); sage; savory; thyme, sweet (tonic); **wintergreen**

SCARS: Cedarwood; frankincense; geranium; hyssop; lavender; myrrh; patchouli

SCIATICA: Camphor; **chamomile, Roman**; **clove bud**; **eucalyptus**; ginger; **juniper berry**; lavandin; marjoram, sweet; **peppermint**; pine; rosemary; sandalwood

SHINGLES: **Clove bud**; eucalyptus; frankincense; **geranium**; niaouli; peppermint; **sage; thyme, sweet**

SHOCK: Chamomile, Roman; mandarin; melissa, true; neroli; peppermint; ylang ylang

SINUSITIS: Basil; bay; cajuput; clove bud; eucalyptus; hyssop; marjoram; niaouli; peppermint; pine; rosemary; sage; tea-tree; thyme, sweet

SKIN, CRACKED/CHAPPED: Benzoin, chamomile, German; patchouli; rose otto; sandalwood

SKIN, DRY: **Chamomile, German**; chamomile, Roman; geranium; **lavender**; **neroli**; petitgrain; rose otto; sandalwood; vetiver

SKIN, MATURE: Benzoin; **clary sage**; **fennel**; **frankincense**; geranium; lavender; myrrh; neroli; rose; sandalwood

SKIN, OILY: Bergamot; camphor; **cedarwood; cypress**

SKIN, OPEN PORES: Geranium; **juniper**; lavender; lemon; petitgrain; rosemary; ylang ylang

SKIN, SENSITIVE: Chamomile, German; geranium; neroli; rose otto; sandalwood

SORE THROAT: **Cedarwood**; clove bud; **eucalyptus**; geranium (inflammation); lavender (inflammation); lemon; lemongrass; myrrh; peppermint; pine; niaouli; **sandalwood** (soothing); thyme

SPRAINS: Chamomile, German; fennel; hyssop; **lavender**; marjoram, sweet; nutmeg (analgesic); rose otto; **rosemary**

STIMULANT: Cypress; marjoram, sweet; niaouli

STRETCH MARKS: Carrot seed; frankincense; **geranium; lavende**r; myrrh; orange, bitter

SUNBURN: Geranium; lavender; **peppermint** (no more dm 1%); sandalwood

SWEATY SMELLS: Cypress; ginger; nutmeg; pine; sage; savory; thyme, red; thyme, sweet

TENDONITIS: Chamomile, German and Roman; frankincense; juniper berry; pine; rosemary

THREAD VEINS: Chamomile, German and Roman; cypress; frankincense; lavender; lemon; neroli; orange, sweet; patchouli; peppermint; rose otto

OVERACTIVE THYROID: Clove bud; marjoram, sweet; **myrrh**

TONIC (CIRCULATION): Cedarwood (lymph); cypress; **orange, bitter**; rosemary (blood); sage; **sandalwood; thyme, sweet**

TONIC (MUSCLES): Black pepper; cinnamon

TONSILLITIS: Clove bud; eucalyptus; geranium; lemon; niaouli; rosemary; sage; thyme, sweet

TOOTHACHE: Black pepper; cajuput; chamomile, Roman (teething); clove bud; ginger; nutmeg; pine; sage

TRAVEL SICKNESS: Caraway; ginger; peppermint

ULCERS: Benzoin; **chamomile, German; geranium; lavender**; lemon; myrrh

URINARY TRACT INFECTIONS: Bergamot; chamomile; eucalyptus; fennel; frankincense; geranium; juniper; lavender; sandalwood; **tea-tree**; thyme

VAGINITIS: Chamomile, German; clary sage; lavender; niaouli (infection); **tea-tree** (infection); thyme, red (infection); thyme, sweet

VARICOSE ULCERS: Benzoin; chamomile, German; geranium; lavender; **lemon; myrrh; niaouli**

VARICOSE VEINS: **Basil**; cajuput; **clary sage; cypress; juniper** (stimulant); lemon; **neroli; niaouli**; patchouli (decongestant); peppermint (cooling); rosemary (astringent); sandalwood (soothing); tea-tree; valerian

VERRUCA: Lemon; thyme, sweet

VERTIGO: **Basil; caraway**; lavender; lemon; marjoram, sweet; **melissa, true**; orange, bitter

WRINKLES: Fennel; frankincense; neroli; rose otto

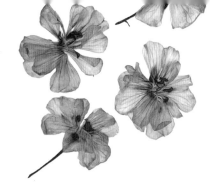

APPENDIX 3

GLOSSARY OF TERMS

Abortifacient: Agent that can cause a miscarriage.

Amenorrhoea: Abnormal absence of menstruation.

Anti-allergic: Preventing allergies.

Aromatology: The study of essential oils for health.

Astringent: Contracting bodily tissues.

Balsamic: Soothing, restorative properties.

Carminative: Relieving flatulence (wind).

Chemotype: Plant grown from cutting in order to propagate plant with known chemical constituent.

Chemovar: Another name for chemotype (var = variety).

Cholagogue: Stimulating flow of bile.

Cicatrisant: Healing, promoting scar tissue formation.

Cohobation: Water used for distillation redirected into system, to be used repeatedly in a closed cycle.

Cytophylactic: Encouraging cell regeneration.

Diuretic: Stimulating the secretion of urine.

Dysmenorrhoea: Abnormally painful or difficult menstruation.

Emmenagogue: Inducing menstruation.

Emulsion: A fluid formed by the suspension of one liquid in another, e.g. oil and water.

Endothelium: The tissues covering the inside surfaces of the body.

Epithelium: The tissues covering the outside surfaces of the body.

Expectorant: Aids removal of catarrh.

Fixed oil: Non-volatile lubricating extract from seeds or nuts, e.g. sunflower oil or almond oil.

Galactogogue: Bringing on the flow of milk.

Hepatic: Tonic to the liver.

Hypatoxic: Toxic to the liver.

Hypertension: High blood pressure.

Hypertensive: That which raises blood pressure.

Hypotension: Low blood pressure.

Hypotensive: Lowers blood pressure.

Hormonal: Balances (or regulates) the body's hormone secretion.

Immunostimulant: Stimulating the body's own natural defence system.

Lipolytic: Breaks down fat.

Mucolytic: Breaks down mucus.

Nervine: Nerve tonic.

Neurotoxic: Toxic to the nervous system.

Osmology: The study of smell.

Phytotherapy: Use of the whole plant, as well as the essential oil, to aid healing.

Probiotic: That which favours the beneficial bacteria in the body, while inhibiting harmful microbes. Literally 'favouring life' as opposed to antibiotic, 'hostile to life'.

Psychoneuroimmunology: The study of the interrelationship and mental effects of the mind, nervous system and body's defence system.

Purgative: Causes evacuation of the bowels.

Quencher: Quenches, i.e. controls side effects.

Rubefacient: Increases local circulation, making skin red.

Scarification: Making a series of small cuts – a method of extracting essence from citrus fruit peel.

Sedative: Producing a calming effect.

Spasmolytic: Relieving muscle spasm or cramp.

Stimulant: Having a rousing, uplifting effect on the body and mind.

Stomachic: Good for stomach.

Sudorific: Inducing perspiration.

Synergy: Literally means 'working together'; the phenomenon that occurs when two or more substances used together give a more effective result than any one of the substances used alone.

Vaso-constrictive: Causes contraction of the blood vessels.

Vulnerary: Healing agent for cuts, wounds and sores.

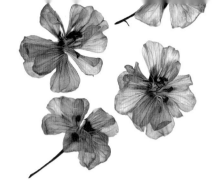

BIBLIOGRAPHY

Viktor Blevi and Gretchen Sween, *The Complete Book of Beauty*, Avon Books (1993), New York, USA.

Jane Buckle, *Clinical Aromatherapy*, Churchill Livingstone (2003), London, UK.

Nicholas Culpeper, *The Complete Herbal*. First published 1653; this edition Wordsworth Reference (1995), London, UK.

Essential Science Publishing (Compiler), *Essential Oils Desk Reference (2000)*, USA.

Ernest Guenther, *The Essential Oils* (Vols 1–6), D. Van Nostrand Co. (1982), New York; Robert E. Krieger Pub. Co. Inc., Florida, USA.

Dr S.K. Jain, *Medicinal Plants*, National Book Trust (1994), New Delhi.

Julia Lawless, *Home Aromatherapy*, Readers Digest (1993).

Dr Vivian N. Lunny, *The Essential Oil Primer* (1993), privately published.

Shirley Price, *Aromatherapy for Common Ailments* (2003), Simon and Schuster, New York, USA.

Shirley Price, *Aromatherapy Workbook*, Thorsons (1993), London, UK.

Daniele Ryman, *Aromatherapy*, Bantam (1993), New York, USA.

Stephanie L. Tourles, *The Herbal Body Book*, Storey Publishing (1995), Pownel, Vermont, USA.

Maggie Tisserand, *Aromabeauty Plan*, Vermillion/Random House (1994), London, UK.

Dr Jean Valnet, *The Practice of Aromatherapy*, The C. W. Daniel Company Ltd (1982), Saffron Walden, UK.

Richard J. Wagman, *Medical and Health Encyclopedia* (Vols 1–4), J. G. Ferguson Publishing Co. (1993), Chicago, USA.

Brenda Walpole, (Vol. 6) *Encyclopedia of Science*, Macmillan Publishing Co. (1991), New York, USA.

Chrissie Wildwood, *Creative Aromatherapy*, Piatkus Books (1994), London, UK.

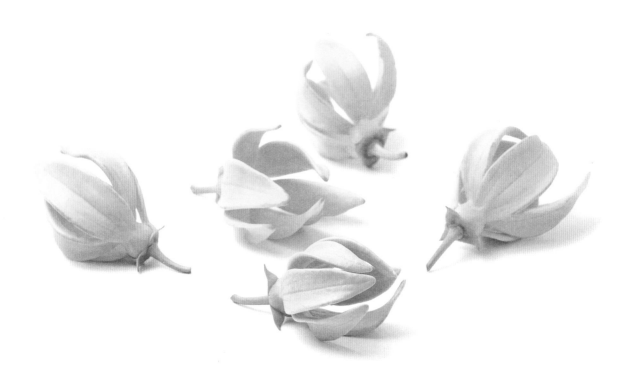

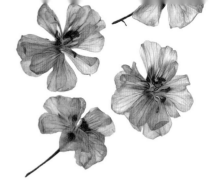

ACKNOWLEDGMENTS

I am indebted to the universal guiding principle, my gurus (teachers) and my parents, who showed me the path of holistic health and healing. The knowledge of essential oils and their therapeutic effects has been revealed to me in a mysterious way. Due to early influence and upbringing in a family of medical professionals, I have always been interested in health and health maintenance. But looking back, I feel amazed at how my heritage, as well as all the knowledge garnered from my studies in botany, zoology and chemistry (including a masters in zoology), and my professional experience as a perfumier, all combined to lead to the field of aromatherapy. I believe it shows the plan of the universe to prepare me for the understanding of aromatherapy.

The support, push and feedback from Minoo, my wife, a practising psycho-aromatherapist who always demands the best possible formulations for her clients, led me to innovate combinations of oils and their usage, which I have shared in this book. I am thankful to Minoo and my daughters Vartika and Kartikeya for their support of and patience with me.

I am also thankful to all my students and workshop participants (primarily health and beauty therapists) for enriching my knowledge through various interactions. Truly, teaching is the way of learning. I would also like to offer my gratitude to all the authors, whose names are given in the bibliography, who have acted as my teachers; each one has contributed to my knowledge in the field.

A book is the result of teamwork, and I would like to acknowledge my co-workers and staff for all their time and input.

Also by Dr Ravi Ratan ...

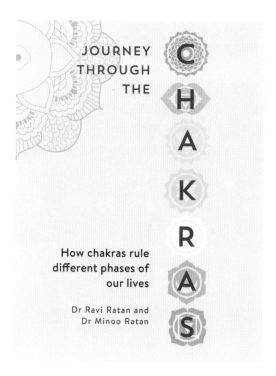

JOURNEY
THROUGH
THE

How chakras rule
different phases of
our lives

Dr Ravi Ratan and
Dr Minoo Ratan

ISBN: 978-1-925682-99-1

Journey Through the Chakras is a comprehensive guide to the inner workings of the chakra system from an age-old Indian spiritual, metaphysical and tantric perspective.

The book dives deep into one of the most ancient structures of the spiritual body. With both anatomical and physiological views, it deconstructs the complexities behind the system, explaining the chakras in a simple fashion that is accessible to anyone.

Available at all good book stores or online at rockpoolpublishing.co

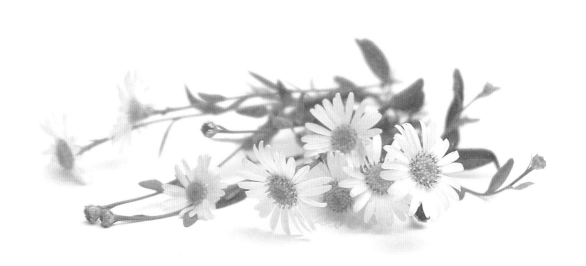